The Web of Inclusion
Faculty Helping Faculty

Patricia Bayles, MN, RN,
and
Jodi Parks-Doyle, EdD, RN
Editors

National League for Nursing Press • New York
Pub. No. 14-2682

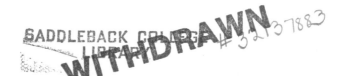

Copyright © 1995
National League for Nursing
350 Hudson Street, New York, NY 10014

> The views expressed in this book reflect those of the
> authors and do not necessarily reflect the official views
> of the National League for Nursing.

ISBN 0-88737-642-8

This book was set in Garamond by Publications Development Company, Crockett,
Texas. The editor was Maryan Malone. The designer was Allan Graubard. The
printer was Clarkwood Corp. The cover was designed by Lauren Stevens.

Printed in the United States of America.

Contents

Part I: Celebrating Our Roots, Exploring Our Present, and Projecting Our Future

Part II: Faculty Collaboration: New Ways to Share Expertise

Editors of Book

Patricia Bayles, MN, RN
Dean of Nursing/Allied Health/
Child Care
Butler County Community College
El Dorado, Kansas

Jodi Parks-Doyle, EdD, RN
Director, Division of Nursing
St. Petersburg Junior College
St. Petersburg, Florida

Contributors

Phyllis Augspurger, MSN, RN
Nursing Department
Xavier University
Cincinnati, Ohio

Jeanette. C. Bernhardt, PhD, RN
Chairman, Professor of Nursing
West Georgia College
Department of Nursing
Carrollton, Georgia

Mary Jo Boyer, RN, DNSc.
Associate Dean and Director
Allied Health and Nursing
Delaware County Community
College
Media, Pennsylvania

Joyce C. Cicco, MSN, RN, CS
Professor
Butler County Community
College
Butler, Pennsylvania

Sandra K. Croyle, PhD, RN
Professor
Butler County Community
College
Butler, Pennsylvania

Sister Rosemary Donley, RN,
PhD, FAAN
Executive Vice President
The Catholic University of
America
Washington, DC

Geraldine A. Evans, PhD
Executive Director
Illinois Community College Board
Springfield, Illinois

Venner M. Farley, EdD, RN
Dean, Health Professions
(Retired)
Golden West College
Huntington Beach, California

Marian S. Gustafson, MSN, RN
Professor
Program Evaluation Plan
Coordinator
Butler Community College
Butler, Pennsylvania

Marie Guynn, MSN, RN
Associate Professor
Department of Nursing
West Georgia College
Carrollton, Georgia

Carolyn F. Hickox, RN, MS
Assistant Professor
Department of Nursing
West Georgia College
Carrollton, Georgia

P. K. Holmes, RN
Interim Director, LPN Upward
Mobility Program
University of South Dakota
Sioux Falls, South Dakota

Linda L. Hunt, PhD, RN
Director, Associate Degree
Nursing Program
Ohio University—Zanesville
Zanesville, Ohio

Carol A. Ignaczak, MSN, RN
Associate Professor
Butler County Community
College
Butler, Pennsylvania

Susan J. Johnson, EdD, RN
Associate Professor and
Chairperson
Department of Nursing
University of South Dakota

June Peterson Larson, MS, RN
Associate Professor and Director
Department of Nursing
University of South Dakota
Vermillion, Campus
Vermillion, South Dakota

Cheryl Leuning, PhD, RN
Associate Professor of Nursing
Augustana College
Sioux Falls, South Dakota

Maryanne V. Lieb, MSN, RN
Assistant Professor of Nursing
Delaware County Community
College
Media, Pennsylvania

Carol Lindeman, PhD, RN, FAAN
NLN President
Dean and Professor
School of Nursing
Oregon Health Sciences
University
Portland, Oregon

Ouida Anne Miller, BSN, MA,
RNC
Nursing Program Director
Valencia Community College
Orlando, Florida

Marcia F. Miller, MSN, RN, CS
Associate Professor
Sinclair Community College
Dayton, Ohio

Jeanne M. Novotny, PhD, RN
Kent State University: Ashtabula
Campus
Ashtabula, Ohio

Karen L. Rankin, MS, RN
Assistant Professor
Department of Nursing
West Georgia College
Carrollton, Georgia

Linda S. Rieg, MSN, RN
Nursing Program
Xavier University
Cincinnati, Ohio

Lois De Jonge Schuller, MS, RN
Executive Director
Visiting Nurse Association
Sioux Falls, South Dakota

Patricia Seymour, RN, MS
Assistant Professor, Nursing
Co-coordinator, Gateway to the
  Caregiven Program
Kent State University: Ashtabula
  Campus
Ashtabula, Ohio

Susan J. Stocker, RN, MSN
Assistant Professor, Nursing
Co-coordinator, Gateway to the
  Caregiven Program
Kent State University: Ashtabula
  Campus
Ashtabula, Ohio

Verle Waters, MA, RN
Dean Emerita
Ohlone College
Fremont, California

Carol B. Wilson, RN, MS
Associate Professor,
  Department of Nursing
West Georgia College
Carrollton, Georgia

Joanne Witt, MSN, RN, EdS
Nursing Program
Valencia Community College
Orlando, Florida

Preface

"I am going your way, so let us go hand in hand."
—William Morris

In April 1994, in Crystal City, Virginia, the Council of Associate Degree Programs held their annual meeting. The theme of the meeting was, "The Web of Inclusion: Faculty Helping Faculty." We are pleased to have had the opportunity to edit the proceedings for the National League for Nursing Press.

This book is divided into four parts. Part I focuses on the roots of associate degree nursing, the evolving changes, and the challenges the future presents to educators.

Part II focuses on faculty collaboration: new ways to share expertise. As a council, we have made an effort to discover pockets of excellence and to share the innovative strategies with our colleagues. On October 14, 1994, the National League for Nursing Council on Associate Degree Programs made history with the first national faculty meeting ever undertaken. This teleconference was sponsored by a grant from the Kellogg Foundation.

Part III focuses on faculty change, methods to enhance the learning opportunities for students, and unique ways to empower students and faculty.

Part IV presents new settings to teach contemporary nursing care. Education must take place in settings where graduates will be employed. The National League for Nursing supports the need to prepare nurses to function as community-based health care providers in a generalist role, rather than preparing them solely for the role of hospital nurse.

The past two years have been critical years for the National League for Nursing. Patricia Moccia met the challenge and has made the organization more accountable and responsive to the membership. This book is dedicated to her for her efforts to make the NLN a web of inclusion.

PATRICIA BAYLES
JODI PARKS-DOYLE

Foreword

The title of this book, *Web of Inclusion: Faculty Helping Faculty*, is based on the American Indian symbol of the "Dream Catcher." Dream catchers are beautifully designed weblike symbols that are hung near sleeping areas to catch bad dreams in the web while allowing good dreams and visions to flow to the dreamer. This symbol seems an apt metaphor as the council considers its future agenda. These are times which call upon us to dream and create the vision of our future for our programs.

This vision began in 1991, when the membership of the Council of Associate Degree Programs (CADP) began a series of open forums at our annual meetings. As a result, the Council theme and four initiatives for the 1993–1995 biennium emerged. Titled, "Web of Inclusion: Faculty Helping Faculty," the initiatives build on the collective knowledge and experience of council members, and ask members to find examples of and to acknowledge their colleagues' innovation and excellence. In planning the 1994 CADP Annual Meeting, the program committee succeeded in doing just that: finding and acknowledging innovation and excellence. The committee designed a program that highlights both national and local innovations. The keynote, plenary, and special sessions by Dr. Patrick DeLeon, Dr. Carol Lindeman, Sister Rosemary Donley, and Dr. Venner Farley discussed emerging national health care priorities, nursing's vision and position within these priorities, ethical dilemmas which these priorities provoke, and the potential roles for the largest group of nursing faculty (us) and graduates (our alumna) to participate in improving the future for all people. The concurrent sessions, developed around the themes of collaboration, change, and practice settings, demonstrate creativity, innovation, and excellence in associate degree nursing education. The vision of faculty helping faculty became a reality with the 1994 Council Meeting and this publication.

Some say visions are easier to articulate than to implement. Yet implementation of collective visions, those that emerged through the Council Forums, are essential. The ambiguity of our times coupled with health care reform, forces us to teach nursing in unpredictable learning environments, environments where expert faculty become novices as both practitioners and teachers. Since acute care settings—our previously comfortable teaching sanctuary—have downsized, we wonder where and how we will teach the skills and knowledge we hold essential. While we yield to the passing of comfortable traditions, such as the 1:10 clinical teaching ratio, we, the faculty, need to become more effective mentors and coaches for our students and each other. How will we incorporate the clinical learning experience into the mainstream of our programs and how will we teach in these settings? First, we must identify the populations we wish to serve. Then we can prepare graduates to meet these populations' health care needs, offering the full spectrum of services such as health promotion, health education, early detection, specific preventions, and immunizations. A wide variety of settings including rehabilitation facilities, long-term care and nursing homes, hospices, Visiting Nurses Associations, and nursing centers need our graduates and provide valuable learning opportunities. As we plan for the future, we will expand our curricula to address cultural sensitivity, learning over time, management, ethics, technology, and primary care.

As we accept the challenge to navigate these times, to dream our dreams, and clarify our visions, we need to rethink, retool, and leave behind what will not work in the future. Fortunately, our history positions us very well for change. We can accept this challenge with the same energy, creativity, and clear vision that our mothers of invention displayed in 1953. We are the faculty who led the first nursing curriculum revolution with the conception of associate degree nursing education. Together, we can do it again! Remember this Proverb:

> **Go in search of people**
> **Find out what they know**
> **Build on what you learn**

This book, dedicated to all dream catchers, seeks to—build on what we learn from each other and to expand the web of inclusion.

Council of Associate Degree Programs
Executive Committee
1993–1995
Susan Sherman, Chair
Dr. Sandy Bowles, Chair Elect
Dr. Betty Warjowitz
Patricia Bayles
Bobbie Anderson

PART I

Celebrating Our Roots, Exploring Our Present, and Projecting Our Future

1

Second Annual Mildred Montag Excellence in Leadership Award: The Founding Directors of the First Associate Degree Nursing Programs

Verle Waters

*A*nniversaries—whether they celebrate a birthday, a marriage, or a public event, are an opportunity for reflection. We pause for a moment in the headlong rush of time to think about what has happened in our lives as a result of the event being celebrated. The past two council meetings—1992 and 1994—have provided us with two 40th-year anniversaries of associate degree nursing. In 1952, the first programs opened their doors and, in 1954, the first graduates became Registered Nurses. Both anniversaries provide a rich opportunity to reflect on our culture and heritage in associate degree nursing.

In 1992, celebrating the establishment of the first nursing programs, the Council of Associate Degree Programs established the Mildred Montag Award for Excellence in Nursing Education, and made the first award to Mildred Montag. In 1994, the 40-year anniversary of the first graduations, the Mildred Montag award was given to the founding directors of the eight programs that were part of Mildred Montag's "experimental" group. Of the eight founding directors, five were present at the Awards Luncheon to receive awards: Hazel Blakeney, Norfolk Division of Virginia State College; Mildred Schmidt, Monmouth Memorial Hospital; Ruth Swenson, Weber College; Mary Topalis, Fairleigh Dickinson College, and

Eleanor Tourtillott, Henry Ford Community College. Founding directors who could not be present were Mary Mansfield, Orange County Community College; Berenice Skehan, Virginia Intermont College; and Lillian Vosloh, Pasadena City College (deceased).

It was an extraordinary event. The five directors sat, together with Mildred Montag and this author (who had the pleasure of presiding and acting as master of ceremonies), at a speakers' table for the luncheon. A nearby table displayed historical items the five had saved, recalling the circumstances and achievements of the early years: correspondence to and from Miss Montag, testy notes and letters from State Boards of Nursing, program brochures announcing the new program, and wonderful photos of brave and enthusiastic students and graduates.

Before asking each of the five to recall the vivid experiences that marked the early years in advanced degree (AD) nursing, I gave a verbal sketch of the social and economic circumstances which gave rise to the bold experiment, shaped it, and contributed to its astounding success. An understanding of our history offers more than an interesting story; in 1994, as in 1954, health care is changing at a dizzying rate, and the certainty that there must be curriculum change is beset by uncertainty about what those changes should be. The stories of the founding directors, who persisted, believed, and built confidence among faculty and students in the midst of a disbelieving mainstream can give daring and stamina to directors today.

The years following the second world war were challenging— and probably stressful—for nursing leaders. A yawning nursing shortage gripped the country. Magazine stories of the day headlined, "Where are all the nurses?" The federal government even conducted a survey to find the answer. More than one factor contributed to the shortage: Contrary to expectations, nurses returning from the war did not return to work in nursing. Instead, they married and began the baby boom generation. Advances in medicine and surgery and rapid growth in the number of hospitals and hospital beds added new demands for nurses. Enrollments in the diploma nursing school (then more than 90 percent of nursing schools) were falling. After the war, opportunities were increasing for young women, and the arduous and isolated world of nursing education was less appealing than other options. Nursing leaders wanted to find a way to respond to the shortage and, at the same time, to reform nursing education. The emergence of a new form of higher education, the public junior/community college was seen as a possible solution. The National League for Nursing Education (forerunner of NLN) initiated a series of discussions with the American Association of Junior Colleges, finding them equally interested in considering nursing among the career programs that would fit into this new, rapidly growing innovation in higher education.

Things moved fast in those few years—1948, 1949, 1950, 1951. Teachers College, Columbia University, was at the center of nursing; some of the most creative thinking of the postwar period about the nurse's function and education came out of this institution. Mildred Montag completed her doctoral dissertation in 1950. Fully attuned to the issues, needs, and opportunities of the time, she worked out the philosophy and plan for an entirely new kind of nursing program. By 1952, the plan was in operation, and the rest is history.

The full story of those first crucial years of operation is full of drama. Between 1952 and 1955, eight experimental programs were established, and the courage, foresight, and leadership of the founding directors of those programs brought ideas into life and shaped philosophy into reality. Most of them held graduate degrees from Teachers College and all were experienced and respected nurse educators.

As the five who were present at the luncheon told their stories of those early years, the tenacity, creativity, and passionate belief in what they were doing came through. Eleanor Tourtillott recounted her oppressively frequent communications from a nervous Michigan State Board of Nursing and described her patient and gallant responses to many requests. When, near the end of the first two-year period, the Board suggested that they (the Board) would review the records of second year students and ascertain whether they were eligible for graduation, the college president at Henry Ford put his foot down and advised the Board that he was fully capable of determining eligibility for graduation of nursing students and all other students (and had been doing so for a number of years).

A stunning story was fully told for the first time: Two of the directors made dramatic decisions (in one instance, probably illegal as well as dramatic) to integrate their student bodies at a time when segregation was the rule in education. In Ogden, Utah, Ruth Swenson admitted an African-American young woman into nursing, and learned that the college dormitory refused her a room because of her race. Ruth then drove the student around Ogden until they found a room for her in a family home. It was not an easy search, and the host family lived some distance from the campus. Until she graduated, the faculty and her fellow students saw to it that she had a ride each day to campus or the clinical agency.

In the meantime, Hazel Blakeney was starting up a program in the Norfolk Division of Virginia State College, a segregated branch of the college established for African-Americans. A white mother and daughter who lived near the college applied for admission, and were first denied by reason of their race. But they were persistent and kept calling Hazel. They lived in Norfolk, wanted to be nurses, and the new nursing program made the most sense to them because of its length, cost, and availability. Hazel told us that finally she decided to admit the mother-daughter pair; her personal conviction was that it was the right thing to do even though it was against state law at the time. In this case as well, the students were successful.

Although there were nursing leaders who advocated for and supported the experimental programs, the rank and file of the nursing world often viewed the new programs as outrageous, dangerous, and doomed to failure. Each of the directors remembers encounters with disbelievers and hostile groups. They gave tribute to the students in the first classes whose eagerness, achievements, and good humor cheered the faculty and director.

It was an inspiring hour. The eight women who established and led the first programs had the courage and the vision to carve out a radically new concept in nursing education. With no path to follow, they provided the leadership for a movement that would result in the transformation of nursing education. We may be facing now, in the 1990s, the need, once again, for transformation in education.

2

Integrity, Access, and Accountability: Health Care Reform's New Ethical Dilemmas

Sister Rosemary Donley

*M*ost analysts acknowledge that a health care system should allow persons in need to receive basic care at reasonable costs in the most appropriate setting. Such goals are ethical principles or maxims. If a health care system were infused with these principles, it would possess integrity or wholeness, guarantee access to health services, and be accountable to patients.

In his September 1993 speech to the U.S. Congress, President Clinton proposed a plan for health care reform based on six principles: security, simplicity, savings, choice, quality, and responsibility (*Domestic Policy Council,* 1993). The term *responsibility* has now been changed to *accountability* and will be used interchangeably. These principles represent a departure from the previous framework of access, quality, and cost containment that has shaped health care policy analysis for the past quarter century. In this chapter, I will examine the principles, assumptions, and underlying values of the Clinton health care agenda within the framework of integrity, access, and responsibility/accountability.*

---

*The recent decision by congressional leaders not to pursue the Clinton health care reform, or other reform, agendas in 1994 does not, in anyway, ameliorate the necessity for reform.

SECURITY

Security has replaced access in the language of health care reform.
When President Clinton speaks of security, he envisions a system
where ". . . every American would receive a health care security
card that will guarantee a comprehensive package of benefits over
the course of an entire lifetime" (*Domestic Policy Council,* 1993,
p. 108). The term security is being used to mean universal coverage
or health insurance for all. In the United States, health insurance is
a work-related benefit that is not mandatory. Approximately 54 percent of the insured population have insurance as an employee benefit (Connolly, 1993). However approximately 36 million of the 250
million Americans (14.7 percent) are uninsured. What is the makeup
of the 36 million Americans that President Clinton wants to help
(Crawford, 1993)? They may have any one or more of the following
characteristics:

- They are too young for Medicare.
- They are ineligible for Medicaid because their incomes are
  above the current Medicaid/Welfare standards.
- They do not qualify for veterans benefits, CHAMPUS, military
  health care benefits, or Indian Health Service benefits.
- They are not in prison.
- They work in small companies which do not offer health insurance as a fringe benefit.
- They are temporary workers/per diem workers/contingent
  workers and are not eligible for benefits. The labor department
  reports this group grew ten times faster than other employed
  workers between 1982–1990 (Barrier, 1994).
- They elect not to buy into their work-related health insurance
  programs because they do not believe they can afford their
  share of the insurance premium.
- They are undocumented aliens. Their previous experience with
  serious illness has limited their ability to acquire health insurance. In the language of the industry, they have bad experience ratings.
- They or their uninsured spouses are temporarily out of
  work/or have changed jobs. About 100,000 workers lose their

health insurance each month when they lose or change jobs (Rubin, 1993).

- They are between 18 and 22, are no longer covered by their parents' insurance, and have elected not to obtain their own insurance policies.

- They are in one of the uninsured groups and their present episode of illness is not covered by workmens' compensation or automobile insurance.

In the Clinton scenario, these 35.7 million Americans lack security and may be proxies for everyone. Under his reform plan, the uninsured, except undocumented aliens, would have received a health care security card.

Today when the uninsured become ill or injured, they seek care in hospital emergency rooms. They are the faces behind the "uncompensated care." It must be recognized in any honest discussion of the principle of security that the uninsured *do* receive health care. However, the approach of the uninsured to health care services and the care itself are episodic and crisis-oriented, because uninsured persons lack access to primary care, preventative care such as immunizations, pre-natal care, cancer screening, well child care or health screening, and the management of chronic illness. Because the uninsured cannot afford, or do not value preventive strategies, their illnesses tend to be more serious when they seek treatment because they have ignored symptoms and delayed treatment. The uninsured also receive the most expensive health care, emergency room care, in-patient care, intensive care, operating room care, or premature and newborn intensive care.

Often lack of insurance limits a person's ability to follow a treatment plan. One statistic frequently quoted is that 17 million senior citizens do not pick up their prescriptions each year because prescription drugs are not covered by Medicare and they cannot afford to pay their drug bills (Clinton, 1994).

Health security is guaranteed in some countries. All other first-world countries except South Africa have a universal insurance program and all other first-world countries spend less than the United States on health care. In 1989, the United States spent 40 percent more per person for health care than Canada, 18.2 percent more than Great Britain, and 12.7 percent more than Japan (Pan American Health Organization, 1992).

   Possession of a health insurance card, by itself, does not guarantee care if access to care is impeded by geographic isolation in rural
communities or inner cities, lack of a sufficient number of primary
care practitioners, linguistic or cultural obstacles, or ignorance about
available services. Access is a broader concept than security. The
acquisition of a health care security card is not a sufficient, condition for achieving health care services. For persons to have access
to care, significant changes must occur in the delivery system itself.
   Within a political environment, security is a more comforting and
familiar word than access. Perhaps it is too cynical to ask if the dis-
appearance of the concept of access from Clinton's formulation of
basic health care principles emphasizes that reform is about health
care financing and not health care delivery. Or is the choice of
words merely a political effort to make universal coverage under-
standable and desired by voters?

SIMPLICITY

If the parameters of reform follow the blueprint outlined in President Clinton's speech to the governors and to the Congress on September 22, 1993 (Domestic Policy Counsel, 1993), the paperwork
associated with the seeking of reimbursement will be lessened because of common forms. Today it is estimated that 20 to 25 cents of
every health care dollar pays for paperwork and the bureaucracy
that it nourishes and sustains. Former Secretary of Health and
Human Services, Louis Sullivan, projected a savings of $8 billion if
the four billion medical forms generated each year were processed
electronically (Iglehart, 1992). Transition to a common form will not
only lower costs, it will make reporting easier for everyone. President Clinton also thinks that simplifying the reimbursement system
will lessen fraud and abuse. It can be argued that simplicity will
make the health care financing more accountable.

SAVINGS

When the Clintons describe one characteristic of our health care
system, the fact that we spend 14 percent of the GNP for health care
while other countries spend 10 percent or less, they emphasize the
savings in the reform proposal, not the costs of universal coverage.

Health care costs are soaring at twice the rate of inflation. Americans spend twice as much for health care as for defense and education, and nine times more for health than we spend on fighting crime (Immerwahr, Johnson, & Kernan-Schloss, 1993).

Each year workers and their employers pay an average of $5,000 per worker for insurance. Individuals also pay over $2,000 in federal taxes for health care and about $700 in insurance premiums, while employers spend over $2,200 to insure workers and their families (*Condition Critical,* 1992). Health care expenditures explain one-seventh of American economic activity (Rubin, 1993). President Clinton argues that if our country spent less for health care, it would be more competitive in the world market. Individuals would have more money to spend on other things because they would not be paying so much for health premiums.

Why does health care cost so much in the United States? Why can't we be more accountable for health care costs? Are we wasteful? Can the answer be found in analyzing unnecessary diagnostic services and treatment? Are there too many players? The array of 1,500 private insurance companies, Medicare, and some 50 different Medicaid programs each have different rules, deductibles, and forms. Does our fascination with high technology treatment and specialized medicine explain our costs, the $700 a day bill for a private room and the $6,000 cost for a normal child birth? In 1950, cataract surgery as we know it did not exist. In 1991 with laser and advanced surgical techniques, surgeons improved the sight of 1 million Americans at a cost of $3 billion. (*Condition Critical,* 1992). According to a *Wall Street Journal* article, cataract surgery is not as well reimbursed as it was six years ago. Today the average reimbursement for this 20-minute process is $1,150 (U.S. backed agency urges limited cataract surgery, 1993). Are physicians the bad guys? When most doctors finish training, they face, on average, loan repayments of $45,000. The average income of physicians is $155,800. Surgeons average $220,500 a year (Pope & Schneider, 1992). Physician income accounts for 14 percent of what Americans spend for health, $832 billion. Are there too many specialists? Although the supply of physicians doubled between 1960–1990, fewer than 40 percent of the practicing physicians are in primary care (Colwill, 1992). The ratio of specialist to generalist physicians in the United States, although explainable because status and financial awards have encouraged specialty practice, does not match the ratios of any other country in the world (Schroeder, 1992). Is the cost problem intensified by the

aging of our population? Right now people over 65 make up 12 percent of our population although they account for one-third of the
health care costs. Yet Japan and western Europe also have an aging
population and, as stated earlier, spend less for health care services.
Is it a by-product of our drug culture and the violence in our society? Has health care cost escalation been made worse by the AIDS
epidemic and the reappearance of drug-resistant tuberculosis and
other communicable diseases? What part of health care costs are
explained by greed and by the practice of defensive medicine? In the
United States, malpractice claims account for about 1 percent of the
health care costs (GAO, 1992). No other country has such an ag-
gressive malpractice climate. In Canada, an attorney may not accept
a case with the hope of receiving a percentage of an award or set-
tlement (Coyte, Dewees, & Trebilcock, 1991).

In the Clinton formulation, managed care was presented as the
central strategy to increase savings or lower costs. Managed care re-
moves the classic separation among patient, provider, and payor and
integrates the clinical and financing functions into one entity—a
health care plan. When people select a managed care program, they
choose a system of care delivery, not just a financing program. However, in Clinton's scenario, people may also purchase more expensive health care plans or opt for fee-for-service medicine. Each
alliance will be required to offer their enrollees a choice of a basic
managed care plan, a point of service plan, and a fee for service
plan (Domestic Policy Council, 1993). While it can be argued that
managed care will give financial integrity to the health care system,
the political reality is that for the foreseeable future there will be a
variety of health care financing arrangements.

THE PRINCIPLE OF CHOICE

Choice of a health care plan for individuals, companies, and
providers is an attractive, expensive principle of health care reform.
However although President Clinton emphasized consumer choice of
health care plans in his speech to Congress, the Congress of the
United States will ultimately set the decisional framework for Americans. Politically speaking, it appears that the adoption of the single payor system of Canada will not be an option, because adoption
of a single payor system would increase government involvement in
health care and limit the role of the private sector (Renas & Kinard,

1990). Under this rubric, individuals and corporations would pay more taxes but no insurance premiums. There would be little need for 1,500 companies to offer health insurance plans and no fee for service medicine. If global budgeting accompanied the single payor option as it does in Canada, there would be less of a market for high technology and less price escalation.

The choice of the system of health care reform to be adopted, the most critical of choices, will be made by the Congress. It would be enlightening if citizens were real partners in making this macro-choice. It seems, however, that the principle of choice means that all Americans will be asked to select their own health care plan which will be underwritten by their employers (Priest, 1994).

THE PRINCIPLE OF QUALITY

The yet to be answered question is what are we receiving today for our $832 billion. How accountable are we? How good is the care? How satisfied are persons with the care they receive? What can be said about the morale of the providers? What is the relationship of cost containment to quality?

When governments assess quality of care, they speak of outcomes such as infant mortality, life expectancy, and levels of immunization (Department of Health and Human Services, 1992). In the United States, there is also interest in differences in outcomes which research shows to be more related to geographic location and the therapeutic behavior of providers than to the age or illness of patients (Wennberg, 1990). There is also concern about the effect of treatment on quality of life and general well being (Lohr & Schroeder, 1990). This research on quality of care compares watchful waiting, less invasive treatment, and invasive treatments. It seeks to understand as well as measure what patients want as desired health care outcomes (Fisher & Wennberg, 1990).

If we begin with the extant data, the measurable outcomes of health care are less good in the United States than in other first world countries (Shealey, 1986). Canada, Great Britain, and Japan have longer life expectancies, lower rates of infant mortality, and better immunization rates (Schieber, 1990).

Satisfaction with care is a more elusive concept. Most people are able to evaluate the interpersonal content of care but lack access to information that would help then assess its scientific or technical merit, its necessity, or its cost effectiveness. It is proposed that health care reform will remedy this lack of data because all providers will be given grades on a health care report card, and consumers will have information about the quality of their health care services and the performance of those who provide it.

Morale of providers varies in the age of health care reform. Hospital administrators, insurance companies, drug companies, and physicians are wary of the health care reform agenda because they fear the new system will limit their control and income. Nurses, on the other hand, are optimistic because they hope that reform will even the playing field, remove some of the barriers to their practice, and enable patients to receive primary and preventive care. However, they recognize that their practices and job security will change dramatically as health care delivery shifts from hospitals to community-based programs.

Health care reform promises to assure quality by universal access to insurance and by the creation of Health Insurance Purchasing Corporations (HIPCs) or Health Care Alliances. These alliances will enter into managed care arrangements with only those providers and provider networks that show evidence of quality. Evidence about the quality health care providers will be displayed on some type of health care report card. Successful genesis of the report cards depends upon the ability of the health care community to obtain consensus on the measurement and reporting of desired health care outcomes. President Clinton argues that because Health Care Alliances will not be able to choose providers or networks with "low grades," managed competition will lead to greater quality of care.

THE PRINCIPLE OF RESPONSIBILITY (ACCOUNTABILITY)

During his September 1993 speech to Congress, President Clinton reminded his audience that ". . . we are all in this together and we all have a responsibility to be a part of the solution" (Domestic Policy Council, 1993, p. 118). In appealing to a communitarian rather than an individualistic ethic, the President asked that providers (physicians, hospitals, laboratories, drug companies, and lawyers) not take financial advantage of a patient's illness, fear, or lack of information. He also reminded insurance companies that they should not make it impossible for ill persons to purchase insurance. He then invited all citizens to change their ways. Poor diets, unhealthy life styles, violence, substance abuse, failure to exercise, promiscuous sexual behavior, and reckless driving are health care sins. "Responsibility (Accountability) in our health care system isn't just about them . . . it's about each of us" (Domestic Policy Council, 1993, p. 119).

This brief review of the principles provides the conceptual background for the discussion of the new dilemmas: integrity, access, and accountability. My analysis is grounded in the framework of the virtue of justice and the application of three types of justice, (contract justice, distributive justice, and justice as participation) to the health care reform proposals.

Contract Justice

Contract justice forms the basis of American civil law: I do what I say I will do. I will be faithful to my contractual obligations. State practice acts and the public have described and evaluated the behavior of health care professionals in terms of their contractual obligations. Most courts have acknowledged the principle of "Do no harm," and have mediated malpractice claims. However, within the framework of justice, an agreement between provider and patient can convey a more positive meaning that is expressed by the word covenant. Perhaps it is for this reason that physicians take an Hippocratic oath and nurses take the Nightingale pledge. When a person enters into a professional covenant with a patient, the ensuing bond is not a legal obligation but rather a promise of fidelity to the demands of the relationship (Ramsey, 1970; Pellegrino & Thomasma, 1988). Understood in this way, contract justice requires more than a legalistic fulfillment of a contract or an oath to avoid doing harm; it seeks to achieve what is in the best interests of patients. It requires that practice be guided by the patients' wishes to the degree these wishes do not violate the providers' own principles and norms (Pellegrino & Thomasma, 1988). Contract justice demands fidelity to commitments and speaks to the principle of integrity.

Distributive Justice

Because the second notion of justice, distributive justice, addresses access to health care services, it is often evoked in discussions about health care as a right (Brody, 1981; Harron, Burnside, & Beauchamp, 1983). However, contemporary political rhetoric confuses access to health care with possession of a health care insurance card. Distributive justice conceptualizes the spreading or distribution of "goods," as health care, according to principles that are rational, fair, and grounded in an appreciation of human dignity. The expression of distributive justice cannot end with the efficient distribution of health care security cards. As has been noted earlier, access is more than security. Distributive justice requires access to systems of care that actually provide (distribute) care to people. That there is a real difference between access to care and the possession of insurance coverage can be illustrated by examining data that correlate the level of immunizations within a community with the level of insurance protection. These data show that for some populations, especially two-year-olds, it takes more than having the security of an insurance card to achieve access to immunizations (Wagner, Gellert, & Ehling, 1992). Simply speaking, it takes a reform of the delivery of care system so that persons in need of care get needed services from the right provider in the right setting. The actualization of the principle of distributive justice requires real change in the delivery system so that people will receive needed care.

Justice as Participation

The third form of justice to be discussed is justice as participation (Szasz & Hollender, 1976). It can be argued that President Clinton's principle of responsibility (accountability) speaks to this concept. Under this principle of justice, everyone is held accountable for the use of the goods of the health care system. However, justice as participation also requires that patients and families are intentionally included in diagnostic and therapeutic decisions. It demands that health providers listen to what patients desire and value from their health care experiences. It assures that explanations offer information in a manner that exceeds the requirements of informed consent procedures or the achievement of full disclosure so that participatory dialogue encourages patients and families to become active partners in decisional processes. Justice as participation also lessens the power gradients that separate patients from providers, and by doing so, frees patients to become informed participants in decisions about their own well-being. This expression of the virtue of justice acknowledges the dignity of the patient as a person and recognizes that patients have the most to gain or lose in health care decisions. Justice as participation also recognizes that everyone be accountable for the success of the health care episode, and that clear, respectful communication between patients, families, and providers characterize the dialogue (Szasz & Hollender, 1976).

This chapter began with a comparison of traditional health policy goals with the new goals for health care reform. Will we have a system which has the integrity and wholeness to address the health care needs of all? Will a reformed health care system guarantee access to basic services by overcoming professional and bureaucratic protocols and procedures that ration health care to the poor, the elderly and the minority populations? Will it assist persons who are over treated? Will this envisioned system hold each of us accountable for wise choices and the most cost effective use of health care resources? Will it challenge us with the option of paying more in taxes or premiums so that everyone will be covered? Will it call into question our demands for unnecessary high technology medicine and boutique care? Will it bring about an examination of personal health behavior and challenge us to elect more primary and preventative health care services?

This chapter also raises a set of questions about justice. Will health care reform evolve a system that has integrity and guarantees appropriate access to services? Will managed care and accountable health care plans be accountable to clients and all citizens? If you accept the communitarian ethic, or the notion of justice as participation, the answer to these questions depends upon individual and corporate willingness to invest energy and time in understanding the issues and participating in the decisional processes. Each of us has an obligation to participate actively in the process of health care reform and work for a system that meets not only political principles but also the criteria of integrity, access, and accountability. Each of us has the responsibility to make health care reform work.

REFERENCES

Barrier, M. (1994). Now you hire them, now you don't. *Nation's Business, 82,* 30–32.

Brody, B. (1981). Health care for the haves and have nots: Toward a just basis of distribution. In E. E. Shelp (Ed.), *Justice and health care* (pp. 151–159). Boston: Reidel.

Clinton, W. (1994). *Remarks by the President to seniors citizens from Connecticut.* Presented at Slater Hall Auditorium, Norwich Free Academy, Norwich, Connecticut. Washington, DC: The White House Office of the Press Secretary.

Colwill, J. M. (1992). Where have all the primary care applicants gone? *The New England Journal of Medicine, 326*(6), 387–393.

Condition Critical. (1992). New York: The Public Agenda Foundation.

Connolly, C. (1993). Business mandate center of health care debate. *Congressional Quarterly, 51*(45), 3120–3125.

Coyte, P. C., Dewees, D. N., & Trebilcock, M. J. (1991). Medical malpractice—the Canadian experience. *The New England Journal of Medicine, 324*(2), 89–93.

Crawford, J. R. (1993). Americans in need of help: A look at the figures. *Congressional Quarterly, 51*(38), 19–20.

Department of Health and Human Services, U.S. (1992). *Healthy people 2000.* Boston: Jones and Bartlett.

Domestic Policy Council, U.S. (1993). *The President's health security plan: The complete draft and final reports of.* New York: Times Books.

Fisher, E. S., & Wennberg, J. E., (1990). Administrative data in effectiveness studies: The prostatectomy assessment. In K. A. Heithoff & K. N. Lohr (Eds.), *Effectiveness and outcomes in health care: Proceedings of an invitational conference by the Institute of Medicine Division of Health Care Services.* Washington, DC: National Academy Press.

General Accounting Office, U.S. (1992). *Health care reform.* Gaithersburg, MD: Author. (GAO/OCG-93-8TR).

Harron, F., Burnside, J., & Beauchamp, T. (1983). *Health and human values. A guide to making your own decisions.* New Haven: Yale University Press.

Iglehart, J. K. (1992). Health policy report. The American health care system. Private insurance. *The New England Journal of Medicine, 326*(25), 1715–1720.

Immerwahr, J., Johnson, J., & Kernan-Schloss, A. (1993). *Faulty diagnosis: A report from The Public Agenda Foundation.* New York: The Public Agenda Foundation.

Lohr, K. N., & Schroeder, S. A. (1990). Special report: A strategy for quality assurance in medicine. *The New England Journal of Medicine, 322*(10), 707–712.

Pan American Health Organization (1992). *Organizational Health. A North-South debate.* Washington, DC: The Pan American Health Organization.

Pellegrino, E. D., & Thomasma, D. C. (1988). *For the patient's good. The restoration of beneficence in health care.* Oxford: Oxford University Press.

Pope, G. C., & Schneider, J. E. (1992). DataWatch. Trends in physician income. *Health Affairs, II*(1), 181–193.

Priest, D. (1994). Frantic scramble on health care. *The Washington Post,* p. A-1, 8.

Renas, S. & Kinard, J. (March, 1990). Importing the Canadian plan. *Health Progress, 71,* 22–26.

Ramsey, P. (1970). *The patient as a person. Explorations in medical ethics.* New Haven: Yale University Press.

Rubin, A. (1993). Reinvention of health care is key to Clinton's overhaul. *Congressional Quarterly, 51*(11), 595–600.

Schieber, G. J. (1990). Health care financing trends. Health expenditures in major industrialized countries, 1960–87. *Health Care Financing Review, II*(4), 159–167.

Schroeder, S. A. (1992). Physician supply and the U.S. medical marketplace. *Health Affairs, 11*(1), 235–243.

Shealey, T. (1986 May). The United States vs. the world: How we score in health. *Prevention, 38,* 68–72.

Szasz, T. S., & Hollender, M. H. (1976). The physician-patient relationship. From "The basic models of the doctor-patient relationship." In S. Gorovitz (Ed.), *Moral problems in medicine.* Englewood Cliffs, NJ: Prentice-Hall.

U.S. backed agency urges limited cataract surgery. (1993 February 26). *Wall Street Journal,* B6:4.

Wagner, G. A., Gellert, G. A., & Ehling, L. R. (1992). Correspondence. Insurance coverage for preventive immunizations in childhood. *The New England Journal of Medicine, 326*(11), 768–769.

Wennberg, J. (1990). Outcomes, research, cost containment, and the fear of health care rationing. *New England Journal of Medicine, 323*(17), 1202–1204.

3

Vision for Nursing Education Reform

Carol Lindeman

During this past year, in discussions with many nursing faculty across the country, all made it very clear that they are struggling with changes occurring in the clinical sites they use for student learning experiences, with changes in their own institutions, and with changes in society at large. I recall one faculty member who described a late evening phone call informing her that the hospital she used for pediatric clinical experiences was closing that unit. She was told that the students could not return. In the middle of the term and with no forewarning, she had to find another clinical site. Locating experiences in the community was her only hope. Yet she wasn't certain that community-based experiences were right for the faculty or the students. Her story evoked comments from others describing long-term relationships with hospitals that were now changing as hospitals down-sized, closed units, merged, and changed the staffing mix.

Nursing faculty also expressed concern over their student body. One faculty member described her situation this way, "I used to call battered women shelters to arrange clinical experience for our students. Now I call to see if one of our students can use the facility." Other faculty shared their experiences of having a student body in need of more and more academic and personal counseling services at the same time their institutions were cutting those services to reduce costs. One program director explained that she had returned to school to obtain a degree in counseling so she could be more responsive to the needs of the student body.

Most of us can identify with these or similar situations. We find our programs having to change—or at least we are finding ourselves having to do things differently—not because we initiated the change but because of the change in the organizations and events surrounding us. We live in organizations and systems that are accurately described by the word *turbulent.* Can you recall being in an airplane when it unexpectedly hit turbulent air? Remember the sensations in the pit of your stomach? In this country, education and health care are turbulent systems. Smooth air is a long way away.

For most of this decade faculty talked about change. We attended meetings and discussed a curriculum revolution and paradigm shifts. We assumed we would control the change. Today, nursing education is at the breakpoint. We are leaving one paradigm and moving into another. However, many of us do not feel in control. We in nursing, like many others, are moving into an era very different from the past. We spend an increasing amount of time trying to make sense out of what is happening and developing survival strategies. We are being hurried into a new paradigm because of the rapid changes in post secondary or higher education, in health care, in technology, and in the demographics of the population, in the way organizations function, and in society itself.

Higher education is changing in response to the public's concern that costs for education have increased at rates higher than inflation while at the same time student outcomes are poorer. Higher education is having to do more with less and to make itself more relevant to society. Institutions from the Ivy League schools to the newest community colleges are taking measures to increase faculty productivity, reduce administrative positions, create new educational partnerships, scale down student services, take advantage of new technology, and find new sources of revenue. Many are redefining their mission and emphasizing the comparative advantage. Others are reshaping the academic calendar. Faculty that I have talked with tell stories of class size doubling, elimination of secretarial positions, electronic mail and voice mail replacing humans, and the constant push to do more with less. In one very extreme situation, faculty were required to write exam questions on the blackboard because the nursing unit did not have funds to pay for duplication of exams.

A year ago we thought that by now we would know what the reformed health care system would look like. That is not the case. However, in this last year, health care delivery has changed dramatically. Managed care, that is, a prepaid, capitated approach to providing a specified set of services with a specified group of providers and a specified set of facilities to an enrolled population, is sweeping the country. In the traditional fee for service approach, the more you did, the more you were paid. The incentive was to do more. In managed care, the incentive is to do less. The profit margin is increased when less of the capitated fee is used for services. Managed care reverses the process used to achieve a positive bottom line. Across the country, managed care systems are using fewer and fewer hospital days, replacing licensed personnel with unlicensed and therefore less costly personnel, down-grading positions, and reorganizing and eliminating administrative positions. Sweeping short-term cost containment measures are being implemented as administrators respond to an environment of cost effectiveness, great competition, and shared risk. This is certainly not the health care reform we dreamed of.

Technology is changing the very nature of our work quite dramatically. For example, in the future people will not visit a doctor in person. A person needing medical care will communicate with a doctor by electronic mail. But that would only occur after the person used several self-diagnostic kits and software programs. In one scenario, at birth, an individual will be issued a health watch. That watch will monitor vital health data which will be transmitted to an appropriate data base. Advice about health practices and behaviors will be transmitted back to the person. If you need medication, it will automatically be mailed to the person or the individual will go to a machine like a bank machine and insert their health smart card and the medication will be dispensed. With this ever increasing use of technology, tasks performed by nurses and other health care workers will be "deskilled." The assumption is that technology can reduce risk and decision making, with less well-prepared (and therefore cheaper) people performing the work.

National demographics are changing dramatically as well. The changing national demographics are considered the single most dominant factor in the future of health care. There are two demographic changes that I wish to highlight. The first is the aging of America. We know that, in the relatively near future, one out of approximately every four Americans will be over 65. The "young elders" between 55 and 70 are biologically more active and fit than previous generations. The "golden years" seniors between 70 and 85 are the most mobile segment of the population. These two groups of seniors are recovering from episodes of acute illness to high-health life styles. They are investing their incomes in their own health. Americans 85 and older are the fastest growing segment of the population and are at the highest risk for hospitalization. They are likely to experience problems with activities of daily living and are vulnerable to chronic diseases, incontinence, and decreasing mobility. Three out of every four of these elders are women who are likely to be living alone and in poverty.

The second demographic factor concerns growing heterogeneity. Currently, our population is approximately 84 percent non-Hispanic white, 12 percent African American, 3 percent Asian or other groups, and 8 percent Hispanic (who may be of any race). However, between 1980 and 1990, the population overall grew by 10 percent, but the white population grew by 8 percent, the African American population by 16 percent, the Asian population by 65 percent, and the Hispanic population by 44 percent. The distribution of minorities is uneven across states and within states. Currently, Hawaii is the only state where non-Hispanic whites are in the minority, but in the near future the same will be true for New Mexico, Texas, and California. Given the fact that health care administration has been dominated by the white male model and that the health care delivery system has been somewhat change resistant, these demographic trends will challenge the system. Certainly nursing could provide the vision and leadership for reforming health professional education to accommodate these demographic trends. As dramatic as those changes are, the country is also becoming more diverse and polarized in terms of values. In the near future, one out of every two persons a nurse cares for will be significantly different from that nurse in terms of age, ethnic background, or values. There are many implications here for nursing education and nursing practice, especially the frequently overlooked need for inclusion of more non-Western medicine content and learning experiences.

The power base in society is also changing from a generation of people whose values and attitudes were heavily influenced by the Great Depression to a generation of people whose values and attitudes were heavily influenced by the Vietnam War. This generation is characterized by (1) a distrust of government and (2) wanting to assure the value received for the dollar spent. It is a generation that believes in grass roots politics and privatization as means for solving the problems of society. In this era, more and more issues about health care and education will be placed on the referendum ballot. Many activities that were once the role of government will be privatized.

For example, in one state, new roads are built by a private company which then charges a toll for use. In another state, education from K through 12 has been contracted out to a private firm. These trends will continue along with the challenges to give the public the greatest value for the dollar spent—the greatest value as defined by the consumer. Higher education with its academic rank and tenure system is certainly feeling this challenge.

We are working in nonlinear organizations and thinking in nonlinear ways when most of us were prepared to work in linear organizations and to think in linear ways. In linear thinking, problems are viewed as separate. There is an assumption that problems can be solved or fixed. One can reduce a problem to separate parts and then through hard work and intense thinking find a solution. Once the solution was implemented, the problem went away. The broken wheel was fixed. In nonlinear thinking, problems are not viewed as separate. The assumption is that problems are connected; approaching one problem will lead to uncovering others. Problems will keep coming back to be solved over and over. Nonlinear thinking is a stream responding to constantly changing conditions. For example, violence is a social issue that will not be solved through linear thinking. Every analysis of the issue will lead to the uncovering of other problems, and no matter what we do today violence will surface again in another form only to be "solved" again. Many of the issues we are dealing with today are also problems that we tried to solve in the 1960s. They are resurfacing not because our answers in the 1960s were wrong. They are resurfacing again because our world is one of ever changing conditions.

Linear organizations are like pyramids with a leader at the top controlling the vision and direction. They have rules, structures, and solid boundaries. People know where they fit in and how business is done. In contrast, nonlinear organizations are dynamic. Flexibility is critical and boundaries are constantly shifting. Work is done through relationships rather than structures.

This world of rapid change is our reality as we attempt to create a new vision for nursing education . . . and create a new vision we must. That vision must reflect the multiple realities we experience in this turbulent era. After creating that new vision we must be prepared to change it and change it. The era of changing the curriculum every eight years in anticipation of NLN accreditation is gone. The era of a single best vision for nursing education is gone.

What are the survival skills for this turbulent era?

1. Look at this as a time of opportunity; it really is.
2. Create working relationships that produce energy and unleash creativity; give up past boundaries and hierarchies.
3. Use the past as a guiding post but not as a hitching post.
4. Accept the fact that there is no one right answer: There are many good answers.

In addition, this era requires nurse educators to:

1. Change or go out of existence. There is no turning back nor ability to maintain the status quo.
2. Develop a vision of nursing and nursing education that is shared by those in your institutions (academic and clinical) and your community.
3. Critically analyze every assumption and folklore that affects your current program.
4. Conceptualize and reconceptualize every aspect of the program in light of the realities of this era and the shared vision.
5. Become competent in a community-based health care system—*community* meaning where the control is, where the care is given, what the philosophy is, and population focused.

The realities of this turbulent era can feel overwhelming. Yet community colleges and their nursing faculty should move forward boldly. Community colleges have been built on the philosophy of shared vision and accountability to the community. In this sense, they have always had a comparative edge in the marketplace. The challenge to community college nurse educators is to implement that philosophy at the level of the nursing program. Some faculty have been reluctant to give up control of the curriculum or be responsive to community needs. Faculty have not seized the opportunity to serve on boards of community groups or agencies. Those that have know the significant differences they can make when you wish to use those agencies for clinical experiences.

Recently, I read in the local newspaper that one of our community colleges was holding a series of public forums. The public was asked to attend and to give input regarding the programs and activities of that community college. What a wonderful opportunity for that nursing faculty for dialogue with the community. What a wonderful opportunity not to tell the community what you are going to do for them, but to find out from them what they want from you.

You work in organizations where the administration has a community focus. Therefore, you will find great support to accentuate your linkage with the community.

These are turbulent times. They are so turbulent that we sometimes feel ill-prepared to do our work. For an instructor that has never worked in a community-based setting and has always used the hospital for clinical experiences, it is scary to now be charged with using the community for student clinical experiences. It is difficult to find experiences and perhaps even more difficult to find experiences appropriate to beginning students. It is impossible, however, if we do not reconceptualize the learning outcomes from those experiences. We cannot use the same objectives and just change the setting, nor should we.

These are turbulent times. Nursing education is at the breakpoint moving from one paradigm to another. The best advice I have to offer comes from the book, *All I Needed to Know I Learned in Kindergarten*. One of the things I learned in kindergarten is this: if you are crossing the street, it is best to do it holding someone's hand. Changing paradigms for faculty is like crossing the street for a five-year-old. It is best to do it holding someone's hand. And that is what you have allowed yourselves to do with this book.

4

The Web of Inclusion:
Faculty Helping Faculty to Weave
the Fabrics of Our Future

Venner M. Farley

*P*eter Drucker, the acknowledged frontrunner in management thinking, wrote, "We are in one of those great historical periods that occur every 200 to 300 years when people do not understand the world they live in anymore, when the past is not sufficient to explain the future." Marilyn Ferguson, a well-respected, health science writer, has written, "It's not so much that we're afraid of change or so in love with the old ways, but it's that place in between that we fear . . . it's like being between trapezes. It's Linus when his blanket is in the dryer. There's nothing to hold onto." Those of us who live and nurse and teach at this time near the end of the 20th Century are abundantly aware of the truths in both of these statements. Our mission is to continue the radical experiment of making the remainder of the 1990s the decade of the nurse, enhanced by vast changes in nursing education and nursing practice. If this is to occur, the decade must be organized around these characteristics:

1. The nurse will be key to customer defined quality.
2. The nurse will be pivotal in the development of healthy communities and the prevention of disease.
3. The nurse will be at the center of patient centered care.
4. The nurse will be central to the concept of the healing environment.

5. The nurse will take the lead in micromanaging the processes and costs of medical care.
6. Nurses will be recognized and respected as caregivers who are central to the new health care delivery system.

Nurses must be at the forefront during the most exciting era of the health care revolution. It is critical that the web of inclusion focus on our collegiality, our courage, and our charisma in helping each other—the old and the new faculty—to see things that never were and ask, "Why not?"

We are in a time of enormous change. The only thing that we as faculty can depend on is the predictable uncertainty of the future. So, in terms of changing directions: If you sometimes feel in a state of delusion; east of ambivalence; west of denial; south of projection; take a right turn to resignation; and keep going until you get to self-actualization! None of this will be easy for us who are the nurse educators of the present and the future. As the United States moves into a changing health care system with or without federal health care reform, we can count on the building of integrated health care systems, such as the country has never seen. These integrated health care systems will have these characteristics:

- Customer oriented
- Community based
- High quality, low cost care
- Specific population served
- Effective physician leadership
- Innovative financing
- Availability to the entire community.

If this sounds different, I can assure you that it is. We are looking for nurses today who are creative and who can color outside the lines. For those of us who are remnants of the "good old days," I would urge us to remember that the "good old days" were not as good as they were old.

The tenents for the future of nursing in this new health care environment will be based on:

- Achievement of outcomes
- Financial integrity

- Adaptation to change
- Flexibility
- Agility
- Productivity
- Cost control
- Service
- Quality.

Today the nurse working in the hospital setting would concur with this dictum, "You are either overworked or unemployed in hospital nursing today." Ninety percent of the decisions made in hospitals must be made by the people doing the work. Since nurses are the most numerous of all persons working in hospitals, it seems clear to me that 90 percent of the decisions made in hospitals today must be made by the nurses doing the work at the patient's bedside. This is the major characteristic of the dominant buzzword in nursing today—empowerment. It is, however, true that nurses in hospital settings today are overwhelmed by a conflicting dilemma: Availability versus Affordability. In other words, "the old numbers of nurses at the new rate of pay" just won't work.

Another buzzword in nursing and hospitals today is "re-engineering." Re-engineering asks the question, "If we crashed and had to rebuild *what* should we keep? *How* should we do it? *Who* should do it?" In analyzing the work being done at the bedside of patients in hospitals today, restructuring demands that nurses at the bedside ask these three questions:

1. What's being done?
2. Who is doing it?
3. Should it be done?

These questions must be answered in terms of service, quality, and cost. It is especially important that we as faculty in nursing programs, recognize that you cannot restructure the *work* in hospitals without restructuring the *worker* in the hospital. This has special meaning for us as faculty because it means the redesign of the nursing curriculum, so that the student in the nursing program can be restructured prior to entering a workforce that has changed vastly in the last three years. That vast change has occurred because the unit price of the registered nurse in the hospital setting has increased substantially in recent years. Therefore, there will be fewer nurses in the future working in hospitals; and there will be increased utilization of unlicensed assistive personnel who will do tasks that are not cost effective to have registered nurses performing. Management's job in this future will be to get out of the way: This means to remove the obstacles so the worker nurses and the unlicensed assisting personnel can do their jobs in an efficient and quality-focused manner.

The web of inclusion demands that nursing faculty focus on the elimination of the BMW (bitching, moaning, and whining) club; negaholism; and nurse abuse, both in nursing programs and among nursing students as well as among students and faculty. Leaders in a time of chaos cannot be guilty of negaholism and nursing student abuse. That would preclude success in preparing nurses for the work setting today. We need to prepare students for the LEXUS Association:

Loving
Empathic
Xenophilic and
Utterly
Serene

Determining the delivery of quality nursing care in a time of incredible diversity and, quite frankly, in a time of societal chaos, is the mission of the community college nursing faculty member today. We need to instill in our students the thought that they must be able to save lives on entry into practice with very little time and with slim or slender resources. This is crucial because the future for them in health care delivery will be a turbulent corporate environment; a time when there is no such thing as individual job security . . . when the danger exists of the whole organization failing. As Robert Francis Kennedy said in 1968, we must urge our students to understand that "the future is not a gift, it is an achievement." And we must prepare students so that they are able to achieve that future. Those of us who were diploma trained grew up knowing the rules of the game. Those rules were simple and very direct:

- Don't rock the boat.
- Don't enjoy your work.

- Don't disagree with the boss.
- Don't be first.
- Look busy even when you're not.
- Do not be associated with any failures.
- Don't be the bearer of bad news.
- Don't share information with others.
- Complain (BMW).

The rules of the game, thank God, have changed. The rules of the game in today's health care delivery system are:

- Treat everybody with respect.
- Enjoy your work.
- Encourage people to have fun at work.
- Speak with pride about the organization.
- Initiate changes.
- Be a risk taker.
- Bring uncomfortable issues into the open.

The reason for these changes is very simple. We become what we think; we become what we expect; and we become what we say. It is very important for nursing faculty to be down to earth, to be frank and open, to be interested in their students on a personal level, and to be thorough in their follow-through in the clinical and classroom situation. It is extremely relevant to nursing education today that leaders/winners be grown during the educational experience. For that to happen in a nursing program, faculty, as well as mentors, must focus on practice, caring, coaching, and supporting.

I remember Geraldine Ferraro's speech when she failed in her attempt to be elected to the vice presidency of the United States; she said, "We worked hard; we gave it our best; we did what was right; and we made a difference." What an epitaph that would be for any nursing faculty member at the close of the 20th century.

The significance of growing winners cannot be understated. The psychological contract of employment in the United States has changed in this decade. It has changed enormously in nursing: Students leaving our programs must know that organizations are going to be more demanding than ever before. This is a compelling reason to change curriculum. Our students need to know that nursing careers will not be as well specified and secure as they have been in the past. The nurse who is agile and flexible will always have a job but that job often will not be in a hospital setting. The nursing student must leave our programs willing to ask the question, "What am I expected to contribute in return for what outcome?" This is an enormous change from the usual associate degree curriculum.

The integrated health care system of the late 20th and early 21st century will be different from anything you and I have known before. The 21st century will be a time of great change in all businesses or corporate structures in our country. We are leaning now toward establishing this new business environment in nursing and in hospitals and we must have a significant part in it. Trust will flourish in the 21st century; and the elements of business in the 21st century will be dominated by the following characteristics:

- Integrity
- Respect
- Empowerment
- Vision
- Communication
- Mutual sacrifice
- Small budgets
- Conflict resolution
- Humility
- Recognition
- Accountability.

The vision of nursing in this future can be, indeed must be, attractive, inspiring, compelling.

Venues for nursing's practice in the year 2001 will be vastly different from the community hospital we are used to. This means that our choice of clinical settings must include these health care delivery sites:

- Offsite emergency rooms and operating rooms
- Ambulatory surgical centers
- Subacute services
- Alternative therapies.

Additional skills that will be critical to success will include:

- Case management
- Quality benchmarking
- Wellness
- Fitness
- Education, training and retraining
- Telecommunications.

These skills must be considered in curriculum redesigns that we all must be involved in.

Health care reform, with or without a national mandate, will occur state by state if necessary. The issues in American health care reform all involve registered nurses:

- Universal access to health care
- Advanced nurse practitioners as primary care deliverers
- Recognition of what nurses do in health care delivery
- Third-party reimbursement for nurses
- Quality-quality-quality according to the client and family's definition
- Public health initiatives in AIDS, immunizations, wellness, prevention of disease
- Gatekeepers of the new health care system.

If these are the issues that Americans wish included in health care reform, they must be included in nursing's agenda, too, both for the students and for the faculty.

All of these issues are difficult to achieve, formidable to think about, and fatiguing, for those of us who have been around for a long time. To assist you in acquiring the energy necessary for this new period of growth I give you Farley's Rule of Courage:

$$\boxed{30/70}$$

Explanation: At any given time, if 30 percent of the people involved in a change are interested in the change, you can create miracles.

There will always be 70 percent of the people involved in a change who are not motivated, who are not contributors, who do not buy in. Farley's Rule of Courage indicates very clearly that we do not need to wait for them. In fact, we must *not* wait for them. With 30 percent we can create miracles; we can move mountains; we can even change the curriculum. It makes more sense to shape the future than to fight it . . . to embrace economic realities than to battle them. But I cannot promise that every member of every faculty will be willing to make the moves that I am recommending.

Into the year 2001 and beyond, I urge you to be there; be vigilant; be visible; be helpful; be smart; be honest!

Decide what you want, decide what you are willing to exchange for it, establish your priorities, and go to work. Remember, we cannot direct the winds; but we must adjust the sails.

Let me remind you of the words of the British poet Christopher Logue:

Come to the edge,
It's too high.
Come to the edge, I might fall.
Come to the edge!
So they did, and she pushed . . . and they flew.

REFERENCES

Castro, J. (1994). *The American way of health*. Boston: Little Brown Co.

Governance Committee. (1994). *Visions of the future, a briefing for board members, physicians, and administrators*. Washington, DC: The Advisory Board Company.

Maynard, H., & Mehrtens, S. (1991). *The fourth wave: Business in the 21st century*. San Francisco: Berrett-Koehler.

Wilson, C. K. (1994). *Building new nursing organizations*. Maryland: Aspen Publications.

5

Positioning Health Care Programs
for the Future

Geraldine Evans

*T*hank you for joining us as we explore the juxtaposition of massive change in both higher education and health care—a most interesting time in history! Historians tell us we have experienced massive social changes many times over in our history. Peter Drucker, in his book, *Post Industrial Capitalism,* tells us that some of the most notable changes have been the renaissance of the 1400 and 1500s, the rise of industrialism and capitalism in the late 1800s, and now the information age.

It is trite to say we are in the middle of change since everyone says it to the point that we are all tired of hearing it. Possibly we are even somewhat immune to the massive significance change is having on our lives. But, again, I want to focus your attention on change because change in the world around us demands *action.* We are at the convergence of two massive revolutions—higher education and in health care.

Since the early 1980s, when the *Nation at Risk* report was published, we have been under attack by one report and study after another. It is very clear that our nation is not happy with the product of our education system. It is also clear that the higher education arena has faired better than the K-12 system of education as far as public satisfaction is concerned. We have, however, been hit with equally severe criticism regarding (1) the escalation of costs of our services and (2) the relevancy of our programs. Higher education has born the brunt of the attacks when young people have been unable to secure employment after long and expensive exposure to higher education.

Change in higher education has been slow to come. I believe that most of the educational system is still quite unprepared to cope with the speed and scope of the changes that are demanded. And again I believe that, when change has occurred, the community colleges of the nation have led the way. However, much of higher education is still, as one Minnesota senator put it, "one thousand years of tradition housed in a hundred years of bureaucracy," and I might add—a generation of unionism. All of these factors are forces resistant to change and will make the task of meeting the future more and more difficult.

Now we have added another complication. Your involvement in education is with *health education,* and the whole health industry is in massive change. The public is demanding more and better health care at affordable costs—and costs have escalated in an unreasonable way. The Clinton health plan has brought the issue into the forefront of the news on a daily basis, but it has been an American concern for many years now. I am not appropriately sophisticated in the issues of health care delivery to outline the Clinton health plan or to state the benefits and liabilities of it for this group, but I can tell you that, as the Clintons themselves stated at the Annual Grid Iron Dinner, "on page 23,943—no on page 43,395—it says we are all going to die." Seriously, it is clear that whatever plan we finally achieve as a national model, there are several trends that are obvious, including:

1. The emphasis of health care will move from acute care to preventative care. We will spend more of our resources to help our population stay well, in contrast to curing illness after an injury or attack. This should eventually decrease the cost of health care, but will drastically change the emphasis of medicine and the deployment of health care personnel.

   This has tremendous implications on the need for reform in the nurse workforce. There will be less need for the bedside nurse and much more for the primary and preventative care nurse. There will be an increased need for nurses with competence in primary care, public health, occupational health, and home and ambulatory care.

2. The new trends will encourage more nonphysician practitioners. The education systems will need to adapt.

3. Health care will be delivered by a team of professionals, including those with a nonmedical emphasis, such as, social workers, sociologists, psychologists. New team-building skills and attitudes will be necessary.

4. Care will be more community-based.

5. The number of under-represented minorities and disadvantaged group representatives will need to dramatically increase in the health professions. Our society must expand the health care professions to include more people of color and more of our disadvantaged populations. We must be inclusive to be prepared to adequately understand and serve the needs of all of our diverse cultures and populations. Here again, the community colleges have a unique role to play because we are a major access point for many of these groups. Our role in providing *access* and *success* for such students is very important to our society.

6. Ideas and traditions about licensure will have to be revamped. The licensing system, in place now for nearly 100 years, has been successful in keeping quality high. However, it also has become somewhat self-serving to the professions it represents and has created rigid and arbitrary training regulations. Such boards must now address issues of access and cost, as well as quality. It is abundantly clear that personal and professional interests will not be allowed to outweigh public interests.

7. Cost containment will be everyone's responsibility.

8. The rapid change in medical procedures and techniques will demand constant and routine retraining for all personal at an affordable cost.

9. Health care education will demand massive revision of the curriculum and will demand the use of the newest technology for remote delivery of up-to-date education.

Somewhere in the list we moved from an emphasis on changes in health care delivery to changes in education for health care. There is no doubt about it, the two massive movements are intricately entwined and those of us in health care education are in the middle of the fray.

Community colleges now provide a major portion of the nurses and allied health professionals for the health care industry. The National Center for Education Statistics tells us that 54 percent of all health science degrees conferred are associate degrees to students graduating from the community colleges of the nation. The U.S. Bureau of Labor Statistics tells us that the projected growth of registered nurses and medical technical workers (students educated in community colleges) will be almost twice the growth of the general employment growth rate by the year 2003.

The impact of the societal changes on our institutions will be immense if we adequately adapt to meet the needs of our states and the nation. If we do not adapt quickly and responsively, there will be a tendency for large systems and medical groups to grow their own health personnel and to bypass the professional turfdoms of the existing systems. Change in itself is difficult, but this change will be even more difficult because it will demand a movement out of old education paradigms and old health paradigms into new and creative uncharted realms.

The new systemic leadership trends talk about seeing the "big" picture and developing visions for the appropriate future. A word frequently heard and one we are paying more attention to is "interconnectedness." Our world of tomorrow demands an understanding of our own disciplines, but also of the political and social tones of the world around us.

PART II

Faculty Collaboration: New Ways to Share Expertise

6

Designing a Program Evaluation Plan That Complements the NLN Self-Study Criteria: Outcome Collaboration

*Marian S. Gustafson**
Joyce C. Cicco
Carol A. Ignaczak
Sandra K. Croyle

With the current emphasis on educational effectiveness and program outcomes, the key to a meaningful self-study for NLN accreditation lies in the design of the program evaluation plan. Since our nursing program had both a revised curriculum to evaluate and a NLN accreditation self-study to complete, our faculty needed an evaluation plan to provide us with a database that would be outcome focused, comprehensive, and complementary to the newly revised NLN accreditation criteria for associate degree programs.

THE DEVELOPMENTAL PROCESS

With accreditation criteria in hand, we began to plan and develop a total evaluation of our program. Throughout the process, four people were intimately involved in the various steps with one person acting as coordinator. The coordinator laid the groundwork by gathering background information, familiarizing committee members with current trends, and identifying evaluation models that seemed

*The coordinator thanks Nursing Division Chairman Sharon Brewer for her supportive presence and valuable advice in preparing this manuscript.

to work best for our program. We found two very valuable resources in Watson (1990) and Garbin (1991). After reviewing a variety of evaluation models, we decided to use a discrepancy model that we tailored to our program. Our model was designed to compare actual/obtained outcomes to predicted outcomes or standards. The resulting conclusions guided decision making and the development of a prescriptive plan which included a feedback process for reassessment. See Figure 1 for the design of the plan.

Figure 1. Design of Program Evaluation Plan

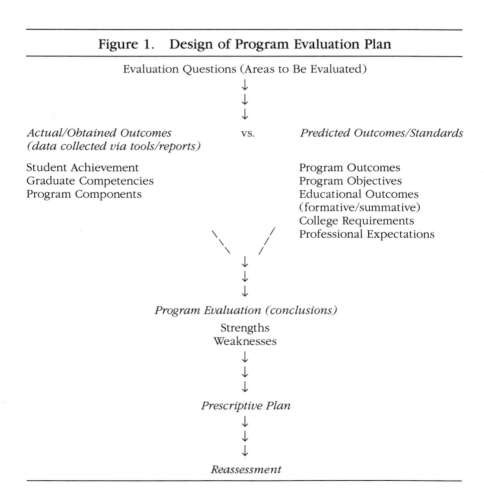

Evaluation Questions (Areas to Be Evaluated)

↓
↓
↓

Actual/Obtained Outcomes   vs.   *Predicted Outcomes/Standards*
(data collected via tools/reports)

Student Achievement   Program Outcomes
Graduate Competencies   Program Objectives
Program Components   Educational Outcomes
                                                                    (formative/summative)
                                                                    College Requirements
                                                                    Professional Expectations

↓
↓
↓

Program Evaluation (conclusions)

Strengths
Weaknesses

↓
↓
↓

Prescriptive Plan

↓
↓
↓

Reassessment

TERMINOLOGY

Much of the terminology was new or at least needed to be comprehended in a different way. After mastering jargon that seemed at first to be foreign, we developed working definitions for words like outcome, objective, educational effectiveness, stakeholder, accountability, and formative and summative program evaluation. These definitions gave the committee a framework on which to build the components of the plan.

The term *outcome* refers to an end result of education. The focus of an outcome is on the aggregate or the whole group being studied. To us program outcome simply meant "what the program does." Our program outcomes were designed to be indicators of achievement of program purpose and were used as standards to identify program effectiveness. Because we also wanted to evaluate events during and after the educational program, we included in our outcomes not only the areas of graduation, NCLEX, and employment as required in NLN accreditation criteria, but also many other areas of achievement and measurements of satisfaction. An example of a measurement of program satisfaction was the desired outcome that clinical sites would report overall satisfaction with their relationships with the nursing program.

The difference between outcome and objective had to be clear. We used the term *objective* when examining individual student behavior after a learning experience. Course objectives and unit objectives were stated to evaluate the individual student in the clinical lab and in class and were developed from the program philosophy. As an example, one of the course objectives for the fundamentals nursing course was "The student as manager of care will use beginning communication skills and techniques." This and all other course objectives were stated at increased levels of performance in each successive course.

Since we described program outcome as what the program does, a working definition for *outcome assessment,* therefore, was a method to know "if we did what we said we would do." Educational effectiveness became a measurement of "how well it was done." We saw our accountability as educators as a responsibility to use the collected information to make decisions that would improve the program or compensate for problem areas that were difficult to change.

When discussing accountability and program evaluation, we had to talk about *stakeholders*—those who were affected by the program and who cared about the program. It is important to include input from all stakeholders when possible so that a broader perspective is gained. For us this included college administration, faculty, students, clinical sites, graduates, and employers. We realized that health care clients were important stakeholders but a complicated group to survey. Equally complex was determining the overall value of the program to the local community. An evaluation of each class related to statistical significance was also needed for program review and future planning.

TYPE OF EVALUATION

When developing our plan, we knew that we wanted to measure achievements and events during the program of learning as well as end results. As faculty members we were interested in determining if the revised curriculum was in need of minor modifications. A formative evaluation provided the necessary data. The NLN self-study required a summative evaluation which included an end-of-program appraisal that would identify program strengths and weaknesses. We decided to organize the plan so both a formative evaluation and a summative evaluation was completed. This meant that separate outcomes had to be developed for each evaluation process. Formative outcomes described the achievement of the students as a group and the program satisfaction of all the stakeholder groups with the ongoing functioning of the program. Summative outcomes described achievement of the graduates and stakeholders' satisfaction with end-of-program results.

An obvious problem with measuring satisfaction within stakeholder groups is that levels of satisfaction will vary based on the perspective of the group and the personal standards of each individual. Even a pleasurable event like spring vacation may have many positive and negative responses when one is simply asked, "How was it?" Comments from students, faculty, and administration would vary greatly. If the concern is whether a week is an appropriate length of time for necessary R&R, then it is more meaningful to ask the question, "How satisfied were you with the length of your vacation?" This will provide information specific to the area being evaluated. Likewise, when evaluating outcomes, an essential element prior to data collection was to clearly identify what was to be measured and what the specific desired outcome should be. Then meaningful data could be collected and compared to the standard.

DEVELOPMENT OF OUTCOME MEASURES

Our first step in developing specific outcome measures was to brainstorm a wish list of outcomes. We asked ourselves questions like: "What would an ideal student, graduate, class, or program be like from the perspective of all stakeholders?" An example of this type question is: "How would an ideal new graduate function?" From the graduate's perspective, it would include being able to report self-confidence in the transition from student to graduate role. From the employer's perspective, it would include reporting satisfaction with the graduate's management of client care in the job setting. From the faculty's perspective, it would include reporting that the graduating class' NCLEX-RN pass rate was greater than 90 percent on initial testing. These were examples of a few of the summative outcome measures we developed. A similar process was used to develop the formative outcome measures.

Our final formative and summative outcome measures reflected the college purpose and the program philosophy and were based on the knowledge, experience, and values of the members of the faculty, college, and profession. Our formative outcome measures were results expected to occur during the educational experience and were divided into three groups: outcomes the student would achieve or report, outcomes the faculty would report, and outcomes the clinical sites would report. Our summative outcome measures were results expected to occur one year after completion of the nursing program. They were divided into outcomes reported by the graduate, the employer, and college administration and data about the graduating class. See Figures 2 and 3 for complete listings.

Included within our outcome measures were the three program outcomes identified as required in the accreditation criterion related to program evaluation. Whenever possible, we used descriptive data, that is, percentages to set the degree of achievement expected for each outcome. As a result, conclusions made in our self-study were supported by statistics. This can be seen in Figure 4, which is a chart we used in criterion 24 of our accreditation self-study.

Figure 2.   Formative Outcome Measures

During the educational experience, the student will:
1. Pass each nursing course with a grade of 2.0 or better.
2. Pass the math competency exam with a grade of 70% or better.
3. Pass clinical with a grade of satisfactory.
4. Score greater than 50th percentile overall on NLN testing.
5. Report satisfaction with personal health practices.
6. Report satisfaction with growth towards the role of nurse.
7. Report satisfaction with clinical progress on self-evaluation.
8. Report satisfaction with overall progress with learning.

The faculty will:
9. Report a class mean total AD score greater than 50th percentile on NLN testing.
10. Report a graduation rate of greater than 70%.
11. Report satisfaction with students; attainment of knowledge of core nursing concepts.
12. Report satisfaction with students' attainment of knowlege of integrated content.
13. Report satisfaction with program's effect on student overall learning.
14. Report satisfaction with students' attitude toward the role of the nurse.
15. Report satisfaction with support services for students in need of remedial assistance.

The clinical site will:
16. Report student competency matches level objectives.
17. Report satisfaction with relationship with nursing program.

DATA COLLECTION

The formative, summative, and program outcome measures gave us very specific criteria to examine. Our data collection tools were developed to be criterion generated in that they focused on collecting data that could be compared to the outcomes. Most collection tools were of the questionnaire type but reports and interviews were also used. Newly developed tools included evaluation of the program by students, faculty, and clinical sites. Some of the tools such as graduate and employer surveys that have been used for years were very

Figure 3. Summative Outcome Measures

One year after completing the nursing program, the graduate will:

1. Report satisfaction with educational experience as preparation for employment.
2. Report satisfaction with readiness for the NCLEX-RN examination.
3. Report satisfaction with attainment of Program Objectives.
4. Report attainment of a job position appropriate for an Associate Degree RN.
5. Report satisfaction with initial readiness for job skills requirement.
6. Report satisfaction with initial readiness to manage client care on the job.
7. Report self-confidence in the transition from student to graduate role.
8. Report involvement in professional activities or advanced education.

The graduate class will:

9. Have an NCLEX pass rate of greater than 90%.
10. Have a median performance within or above the national average in each NCLEX content area.
11. Report employment in a registered nurse position if desired within one year of graduation.

The graduate's employer will:

12. Report satisfaction with graduate's attainment of program objectives.
13. Report satisfaction with graduate's readiness for required job skills.
14. Report satisfaction with graduate's management of client care in the job setting.
15. Report satisfaction with graduate's transition to RN role.
16. Report satisfaction with graduate's involvement in departmental and/or organizational activities.

The college administration will:

17. Report satisfaction with program review results.
18. Report satisfaction from approval/accrediting organizations.
19. Report adherence to administrative schedule for review of documents/services.

useful and helped to support the reliability of our evaluation process. Almost all tools were self-reported and anonymous (except for NCLEX and NLN achievement exams). Validity was supported by utilizing the total population or their mean score as appropriate, by including standardized test results, and by establishing a standard rating scale on all faculty produced tools. All tools and documents such as program policies, curriculum materials, and components within the program evaluation plan were scheduled to be routinely reviewed and updated.

Figure 4. Program Evaluation Results Related to Accreditation Criterion 24

Evaluation Question	Data Source	Program Development	Program Maintenance	Program Revision
Unit in Nursing—Program Function	Administration Faculty		Strength: College & State Board Approval	
Program of Learning—Student Academic Achievement Program Design Comparison with Norms	Students Faculty Clinical Site	Weakness: NLN Basic Nrsg II & III scores Remedial Services Student stress management	Strength: Student academic achievement Clinical Site satisfaction	Content review Investigate expansion of support services
Graduates—Graduate Performance Graduate Role Transition	Graduates Employers	Weakness: Graduate professional activity Data—inadequate on role transition	Strength: Program Outcomes Met: Attrition rate < 30% Graduate rate > 70% NCLEX pass rate approx. 90% Graduate & Employer satisfaction with employment and education	Employer tool—revised to collect data on readiness, management, and role transition

PROTOCOL

Establishment of a systematic format and protocol for this evaluation process was patterned after ideas presented by Bevil (1991). To better organize data collection and to group together related outcomes, we formulated six evaluation questions. They focused on the three major evaluation areas: Program Components, Student Achievement, and Graduate Competencies. Based on the concept of looking for discrepancies between obtained and predicted outcomes, evaluation questions contained verbs such as "match" or "indicate." The core of each question consistently was "Do the obtained outcomes match predicted outcomes?" One example was the summative evaluation area of graduate role transition. The evaluation question read "Do graduates and employers indicate satisfaction with the graduates' transition from student to practitioner in the areas of job skills, management of client care, and professional growth?" Grouped in this evaluation area were several summative outcome measures all related to role transition. Program outcomes related to NCLEX-RN success and employment were addressed in a different evaluation question. Three other evaluation questions focused on formative outcomes and other factors influencing the program outcome specific to graduation.

Each evaluation question was answered by following an established protocol that identified data to collect, tools to use, standards for comparison, analysis methods, timelines, responsible parties, and feedback mechanisms. The process was carried out by the program evaluation committee which consisted of members of the nursing faculty. Although data was collected on a continuous and ongoing basis, data specific to a particular protocol was analyzed every three years. This timing was more effective in revealing trends and relationships.

Evaluation reports included significant data, analysis, conclusions, and committee recommendations. The analysis identified if data obtained was in agreement with the desired standard, policy, or outcome and identified significant areas of similarity and differences. A program strength was indicated when obtained data matched desired outcomes. When large numbers of responses were examined, 75 percent or more of responses per item had to be in agreement to indicate a strength. When comparing one class to another class, mean responses were used. A program weakness was indicated when there was lack of agreement or when 50 percent or less of responses were in agreement with the standard.

The committee made recommendations to the Nursing Division Chairman and Nursing Faculty Organization (NFO). After the NFO discussed the evaluation results, a prescriptive plan was formulated to make program revisions or to guide further investigation of areas identified as weaknesses. A report of action was recorded in the NFO minutes. Specific areas were scheduled for reassessment by the committee one year after the prescriptive plan was implemented. The next evaluation report would include reassessment of areas previously identified as weaknesses and would identify significant new data, analysis, and recommendations. This feedback loop was an essential element to assure accountability.

APPLICATION OF EVALUATION FINDINGS
IN THE SELF-STUDY

The semester before our self-study for NLN accreditation, we completed all six evaluation protocols. Since this was the initial implementation of the plan, newly developed tools were pilot tested prior to use. Emphasis was placed on available data from the classes graduating since our curriculum revision. This gave us a total, comprehensive evaluation of our program. Most data in the report was presented in tabular form to simplify review by faculty. It was a formidable task but it was also an opportunity to examine the evaluation plan, collection tools, and procedures for inconsistencies or areas in need of improvement. One result was the development of a reporting format for the program evaluation committee to use that facilitated recordkeeping. Committee recommendations and prescriptive plans developed by faculty were documented and became an integral part of supporting data in our self-study. In particular, in the Seventh Edition (Rev.) (1991) accreditation criteria numbered 1, 3, 4, 5, 6, 17, 20, and 24 required evidence demonstrating congruency with program outcomes.

Criterion 24 asked that we examine our program evaluation findings regarding the unit in nursing, the program of learning, and the graduates. It also required demonstration of how this information was used for the development, maintenance, and revision of the program or program outcomes. Using our evaluation findings we were able to show that areas identified as program strengths justified program maintenance and areas identified as program weaknesses lead to program development or revision. Figure 4 shows a chart depicting the relationship of program evaluation results to the accreditation criterion.

CONCLUSION

We accomplished much and gained many insights during the entire process. Two factors greatly facilitated the success of our project. We were able to obtain grant funding which permitted a small motivated group of faculty members to work over short but intense periods of time without other work-related obligations. We also received from members of the college administration and in particular from our nursing division chairman a sense of confidence in our work and a belief in the value of the project. The enthusiasm and satisfaction of the committee spread to the total nursing faculty empowering them to see the interdependence of each aspect of our educational program and to use critical thinking to improve and to validate quality within our nursing program.

Our program evaluation plan was one of the many things that made for a smooth and successful accreditation process. We believed that we had a plan that systematically monitored our program's efficiency and effectiveness and would continue to supply data appropriate for accreditation reviews in the future.

REFERENCES

Bevil, C. (1991). Program evaluation in nursing education: Creating a meaningful plan. In M. Garbin (Ed.), *Assessing educational outcomes* (Chap. 3). New York: National League for Nursing Press.

Garbin, M. (Ed.). (1991). *Assessing educational outcomes.* New York: National League for Nursing Press.

National League for Nursing. (1991). *Criteria and guidelines for the evaluation of associate degree programs in nursing, 7th ed. rev.* New York: National League for Nursing Press.

Watson, J., & Herbener, D. (1990). Assessing educational outcomes. *Journal of Advanced Nursing, 15,* 316–323.

7

Mentoring: Making a Difference in Nursing Education

Maryanne V. Lieb

THE HISTORY OF MENTORING

Mentoring is a vital role for nursing and nurse educators to embrace. Although not new, it is just now receiving widespread and well-deserved attention. Mentoring has existed for centuries. Craftsmen, musicians, and writers have traditionally worked under the guidance of a master or mentor. Business executives have also credited mentors for having a positive influence on job advancement and satisfaction. Anne Sullivan, Helen Keller's mentor, helped her achieve her highest potential. This is the fundamental goal of mentoring.

Mentoring also has a history in nursing. Florence Nightingale cites several individuals who influenced her to pursue nursing, but reserves the appellation "mentor" for Sir Sidney Herbert. Herbert, the then Secretary of State in the British army, was responsible for sending Florence Nightingale to the Crimean War where he placed her in a supervisory capacity. Upon return from the war, this relationship continued as Nightingale frequently contacted Herbert for career advice. Linda Richards, another nurse leader, credits a head nurse with whom she worked as mentor—someone who took a personal interest in her career. More recently, 83 percent of nurses polled stated that they have been influenced by a mentor at some point in their careers (Fields, 1991).

THE MENTORING RELATIONSHIP

A mentoring relationship cannot exist without the cooperation of two individuals, a mentee and mentor. The mentee is the novice or "new kid on the block;" someone new to a career or to a particular position within that career. The mentee has everything to gain from this relationship yet the cost to the mentee is minimal. The mentee must only adapt to being the novice which can at times mean sacrificing a certain amount of professional independence.

The mentor, on the other hand, is defined according to the many different roles performed by individuals in this position. The mentor, in most instances, responds to the needs of the mentee, acting in a variety of ways:

- Advisor
- Communicator
- Counselor
- Experienced Role Model
- Encourager
- Friend
- Guide
- Nurturer
- Protector
- Resource Person
- Sponsor
- Supporter
- Teacher

The mentor must be honest, confident, and deserving of respect. A mentoring relationship cannot be mandated; for a successful relationship to evolve, the mentor must also be a willing participant.

The mentoring relationship may be rekindled at any point or may last for years. Mentoring is marked by reciprocal learning. We all have areas of strength; the mentor works to nurture these areas so that the mentee can become the best person possible, both professionally and personally. Frequently the areas in which the mentee excels are different from those of the mentor, which leads to sharing of ideas and mutual growth. This is the sign of a truly successful mentoring relationship.

MENTORING IN NURSING

"In times of change, the learner inherits the earth and the learned find themselves beautifully equipped to deal with a world that no longer exists" (Caine, 1990). This quote signifies how crucial formalized mentoring is in nursing today. With the many changes taking place in the health care world, nurses must strive to help each other adapt. One way to achieve this is for nurses to assume whatever role is appropriate for them at a given time. For example, an experienced nurse administrator is equipped to mentor an individual in administration but may need to be mentored in the area of community health. Fluctuating between the positions of mentor and mentee is expected and encouraged to promote continued growth.

All nurses, no matter what the level of experience, will perceive a certain degree of "reality shock" after making a position change. Marlene Kramer states that this is particularly true when an individual makes the transition to becoming a nurse educator (Locasto, 1989). Kramer's research reveals that there are three phases of reality shock through which a novice progresses. The first is the Honeymoon Phase. During this phase, the educator strives to be the very best, functions with unending patience for all students and knows that they will be as enthusiastic to learn as she is to teach. Faculty committee meetings are thrilling as she watches the more experienced faculty at work; the elimination of weekend and night duty assures a perfect work schedule and just the title "faculty" itself provides a tremendous sense of pride.

Phase one ends and is followed by phase two—Shock and Rejection. There are four characteristics of this phase: Outrage, Rejection, Fatigue, and Perceptual Distortion. The flexible schedules are, at times, hard to handle and the paperwork brought home at the end of the day becomes overwhelming. The novice longs for the seven to three shift when the work day really ends at the completion of a shift. Faculty meetings are frequently scheduled at inconvenient times and require hours to transcribe minutes. Extensive preparation is necessary for class lecture and test construction, yet there are questions the faculty member is unable to answer and unclear test questions. The novice perceives that the job is not all what it seemed and will quickly become disenchanted if phase three, or Recovery, is not actively pursued.

Phase three involves decreasing job-related tension. This can be accomplished by drawing on one's sense of humor and placing aspects of the job in proper perspective. Kramer suggests that one very effective way of helping an individual achieve Recovery is through a mentoring relationship.

AN EXAMPLE OF MENTORING

The mentoring program at Delaware County Community College (DCCC) was begun to ease the transition of part-time faculty into their new roles as educators. A total quality approach was utilized throughout the development process. In 1988, data was collected from the part-time faculty in the areas of educational preparation and specialty. The results revealed that although 90 percent were master's prepared, only 12 percent of those had nursing education as their focus. The need to act on this information was apparent. We realized that our pool of part-time faculty were a valued group of expert clinicians. We also realized that because of the lack of formal education in the art of teaching, they could become unnecessarily frustrated or develop inconsistencies within the program.

The Mentorship Program at DCCC was begun in the Fall of 1989. The group of mentors included full-time faculty and three seasoned part-time faculty, all of whom volunteered for the position. Mentees were then assigned to mentors who were teaching in the same course. Mentors were requested to make a personal contact with their mentee and assist them whenever needed. Mentees were also encouraged to contact their mentor throughout the semester as needed. These guidelines were purposely very general to help meet the individualized needs of the novice.

After the first semester of implementation, both parties were asked for specific evaluation feedback. The mentees stated that what they liked best about the program was having a peer assigned especially to help them individually, their more frequent contact with full-time faculty, and the support network which the program provided. The mentors were pleased with the program but suggested that more specific guidelines be provided to help direct the mentors, that new full-time faculty be included in the group of mentees, and mentors be assigned to mentees who would be practicing in the same clinical facility. All of these suggestions were acted upon. The more specific guidelines provided to the mentors included:

- Make a personal contact with the assigned mentee.
- Call the mentee weekly for the first three weeks of the course.
- Remind the mentee of upcoming planning or course meetings.
- Notify the mentees of what occurred at the course meeting if they were not able to attend.

ANALYZING THE DATA ON MENTORING

Upon completion of the second semester, a new survey was developed and utilized for the following two years. The survey was designed to provide data indicative of the program's effectiveness. Mentees were asked to respond to several job-related areas:

- Having an assigned mentor.
- Having regular contacts with a mentor.
- Feeling confident regarding job responsibilities.
- Having a peer resource person.
- Receiving information about classroom and clinical progression.
- Receiving help when grading written assignments.
- Receiving assistance to resolve clinical issues.
- Feeling a part of the nursing program and college community.

They were directed to indicate how important these areas were to them and their level of satisfaction with each area. The role of the mentor in achieving this level of satisfaction was also explored. The data was then analyzed for both satisfaction and importance (Figure 1). The vertical placement of data indicates importance whereas the horizontal placement indicates satisfaction.

The Fall 1990 data revealed that satisfaction was perceived by respondents in all areas and that all areas except two were felt to be important (Figure 2). Items K and J, which dealt with receiving help when grading written assignments, fell in the lower right quadrant. This meant that even though the respondents did not think these particular areas were very important, they were still satisfied with

Figure 1. Analyzing Mentor/Mentee Relationships

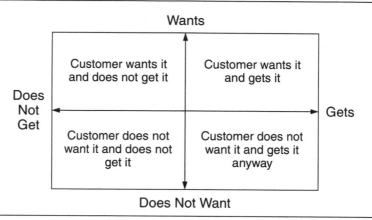

the assistance they received. Item F, which falls at the highest vertical position, indicates that the respondents felt the most important factor was having a resource person available to answer questions and provide support. Item G, which falls furthest to the right, indicated that the respondents were most satisfied with having a peer as their resource person.

Figure 2. Mentorship Program Evaluation: Fall 1990

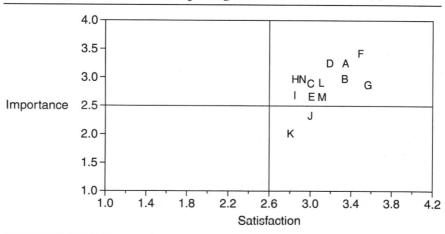

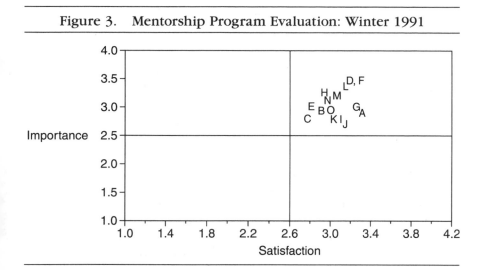

Figure 3.   Mentorship Program Evaluation: Winter 1991

The Winter 1991 data reflected that all areas were again perceived as important and that the respondents experienced satisfaction in these areas as well. The item of greatest importance was again F and also D, feeling confident regarding the understanding of job responsibilities (Figure 3).

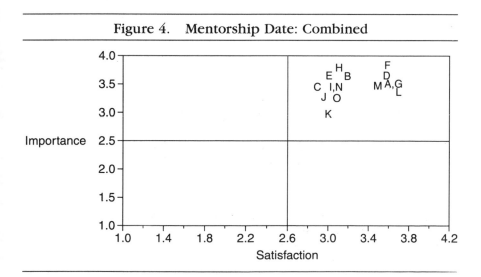

Figure 4.   Mentorship Date: Combined

The Fall 1991 and Winter 1992 data were combined. All items appeared in the right upper quadrant indicating both importance and satisfaction (Figure 4).

The Fall 1992 data was analyzed a bit differently in an effort to identify the mentor's role in promoting satisfaction in their mentee. The respondents were placed into two groups depending on how items a, b, and c on the survey were answered. Those who indicated satisfaction with their particular mentor by marking a 1 or 2 in these items were placed into the satisfied group. Anyone answering these items with a 3 or 4 were placed into the dissatisfied group (Figure 5). The results clearly indicated that an active mentor was crucial to the transition of the new faculty member. All items from the satisfied group (see Figure 6) appeared in the right upper quadrant. Although all items from the dissatisfied group appeared at the top of the graph, indicating importance, the greater majority of the items fell to the left of the midline indicating dissatisfaction (Figure 7). A t-test was conducted with the data from the two groups and reflected a significant difference in the responses at $p = <.05$.

Figure 5.   **Mentorship Program Evaluation Form**

DELAWARE COUNTY COMMUNITY COLLEGE
Mentorship Program Evaluation Form

The rating system is as follows:

4 - Very Important	4 - Very Satisfied
3 - Important	3 - Satisfied
2 - Somewhat Important	2 - Somewhat Satisfied
1 - Not Important	1 - Not Satisfied

Please rate each of the following statements on its importance to you and on your satisfaction with whether the objective was met.

Importance   Satisfaction

1 2 3 4   a. being provided with a mentor   1 2 3 4
1 2 3 4   b. being contacted by your mentor   1 2 3 4
1 2 3 4   c. having contact maintained throughout   1 2 3 4
              the semester

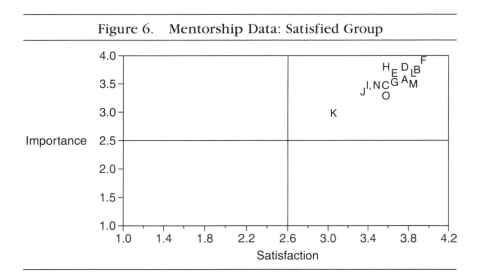

Figure 6. Mentorship Data: Satisfied Group

The faculty at DCCC are very proud of the Mentorship Program. Currently, 13 of 14 full-time faculty volunteer to participate and have identified several advantages from their standpoint. In addition to helping faculty get to know each other, mentoring provides an avenue for the communication of accurate information, promotes

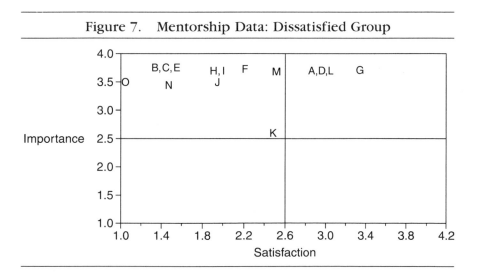

Figure 7. Mentorship Data: Dissatisfied Group

continuity of the program, eases the adjustment of new faculty, and helps the mentor grow as a nurse, educator, and person. Disadvantages identified by faculty mentors included difficulty reaching the mentees and time, the biggest cost to the mentor if one is to be effective.

CONCLUSION

Many of the roles performed by mentors are identical to those of a nurse. Nurses are capable of making a difference in the lives of other nurses as they do in the lives of their clients. The need for mentoring in nursing is pressing and the resources plentiful, if we have the desire.

REFERENCES

Butler, M. J. (1989). Mentoring and scholarly productivity in nursing faculty. *Dissertation,* West Virginia University.

Caine, R. M. (1990). Mentoring: Nurturing the critical care nurse. *Focus on Critical Care.* December.

Fields, W. L. (1991). Mentoring in nursing: A historical approach. *Nursing Outlook.* November/December.

Fox, V. J., & Rothrock, J. C. (1992). The mentoring relationship. *AORN Journal.* November.

Locasto, L. W. (1989). Reality shock in the nurse educator. *Journal of Nursing Education.* February.

Mauksch, I. G. (1982). The socialization of nurse faculty. *Nurse Educator.* July/August.

8

Leadership and Collaboration: Sharing of Power

Mary Jo Boyer

*I*t is my hope that nursing leaders can understand the limitations and inherent failures of the Traditional Management Paradigm. A collaborative approach to leadership is called for; one that empowers others to use their skills and talents for self-actualization, goal achievement, and career development. For this to happen, one must understand why the Traditional Management Paradigm cannot work; why its basic tenets support system failure.

TRADITIONAL MANAGEMENT PARADIGM

The majority of today's nursing educators who are currently in leadership positions probably bring 10 to 20 years of management experience to their jobs. One can assume that their careers began in acute care settings where RNs learned to manage systems and personnel using traditional management styles taught and supported by a male-dominated model of superiority versus inferiority. Nursing leaders learned how to tell people what to do, be in charge, manage tasks, and supervise those who reported to them. Nurses were commended, rewarded, and promoted for this type of management. They were mentored to manage this way and quickly embraced the style and rewards of a system that paid homage to the Powerful Ps: Power, Position, Possession, and Promotion. And what happened? Everyone burned out!

Why did we burn out? For one major reason: It is impossible for one individual, one manager (Dean, Director, Chair), to understand

the day-to-day operational needs of those who are on the front line
with students. We are working with the most culturally diverse
group of students, patients, and faculty that we have ever encountered. We are modifying instructional delivery based on individual
learning styles and computer-assisted learning. We are cruising
along a road that has become an information superhighway. We are
in an era where rapid change, external to education, is impacting on
education faster than we can respond. It is essential that decision
making be diffused among those who are closest to the issues.

COLLABORATIVE LEADERSHIP PARADIGM

I am suggesting a Collaborative Leadership Paradigm similar to the
model I use at Delaware County Community College (DCCC) (see
Figure 1). With this model, the leader is not in the picture; the
leader is on the sidelines, coaching the team to work together. The
Collaborative Leadership Paradigm requires a leader to:

- Promote collaborative decision making,
- Promote interdependence among people who are managing
  tasks,
- Promote teamwork,

Figure 1.   Collaborative Leadership Paradigm

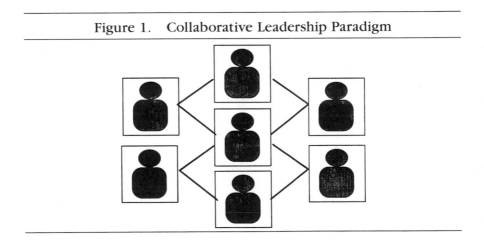

- Influence people's decision making, to listen and give feedback, and
- Step back and be a coach.

Let me share three examples of how I have used this model to effect change, to help my faculty and staff be the best they can be, and to deliver quality services to students in a cost-effective way. The three examples are the faculty travel budget, the instructional supply budget, and full-time faculty reassignments.

The Faculty Travel Budget

Faculty have an established fund to support travel for professional development conferences. The college procedure required faculty to submit their travel requests to me, and I would approve/disapprove the request based on criteria I had established: resource availability, value of the conference to the department, and fairness of the frequency of travel among faculty. This process was fraught with faculty dissatisfaction. Someone was always complaining that someone else has traveled farther or more frequently or used more than their share of the allocated monies. Negativism prevailed and the process created a "we-they," adversarial relationship between faculty and administration.

Using the Collaborative Leadership Paradigm, the faculty now submit travel requisitions to a nursing faculty committee which approves/disapproves each request based on criteria they have established. The committee keeps their own ledger and files an annual report to the nursing department. Any disagreements are handled at the peer level by the committee. This process takes me out of the managerial role and puts the faculty in charge of managing their own system. I have not agreed with all of their decisions, but I do not communicate my disagreements to them. I step back and empower them to take full responsibility for their decisions, successes, and failures.

The Instructional Supply Budget

The department of nursing is allocated $5,000 per year for instructional supplies. Until several years ago, faculty would submit requests for supplies to me on an as-needed basis throughout the year. This system created turf battles between faculty who ordered large quantities for their specific level or team early in each semester. By mid-February, the fund would be depleted. Some teams would get less than they needed to deliver instruction and other teams would not get anything. Again, faculty who were angry at the system blamed me rather than their peers for the inequities that occurred. In reality, all I did was sign off on the release of monies. I had little knowledge about specific team needs because each faculty member/team felt her/their needs were of the utmost priority.

Several years ago, I turned the system over to the faculty. They meet every year in April and determine their instructional supply needs, based on curricular demands, for the next academic year. They use a standard form that lists all equipment, audiovisuals, and computer supplies. They also prioritize their large equipment needs. They submit a formal request to me in May before they leave for the semester. Therefore, I can start ordering supplies in July when the new fiscal year begins. Faculty then have what they need to begin instruction in September.

Full-Time Faculty Reassignments

In September 1993, the nursing department at DCCC introduced a revised nursing curriculum that provided for the integration of Obstetrics (OB) and Pediatrics into medical-surgical nursing. With this change, an OB and Pediatric tenured faculty member, each employed more than 15 years at the college, now had to teach one semester in the medical-surgical clinical area. Both were very concerned about their ability to function safely in a new clinical setting. I could have just made their assignments and required them to update their skills over the summer. This approach would have been consistent with a Traditional Management Paradigm.

However, I chose to employ a more collaborative approach to leadership. I asked each person to design her own retraining program and released her from her clinical responsibilities for an academic semester. Each chose one or more clinical buddies (other tenured faculty members or clinical practitioners) to work with in the acute care setting. Every week, for one semester, both individuals spent their clinical time with their buddy on a new clinical area.

It cost the college $3,000 to hire part-time faculty to replace them in the clinical area. However, it was a small investment which yielded valuable results. Two full-time faculty members were supported by the college and retrained according to their own personal action plans. Each became self-accountable for her new responsibilities. The process was not characterized by anger, blame, or negativism. The only initial barrier that had to be overcome was the mindset of other full-time faculty who felt they would be doing more or working harder than their peers.

BARRIERS TO THE COLLABORATIVE
LEADERSHIP PARADIGM

Three barriers that I encountered when implementing the Collaborative Leadership Paradigm will be discussed next. Some suggestions for ways to overcome these barriers are included.

Administrative Peers

Administrators that are comfortable with the Traditional Management Paradigm will not be supportive of your efforts to use a collaborative model. Managers are afraid to lose power, self-esteem, and possibly their jobs.

Improvement Strategy

Ask a member of the resistance movement to become a part of a team that is working on a project where the collaborative paradigm is being used. Choose a project that is simple and has a high probability of success. When the team is successful and wins praise, step back and let others take the praise, especially anyone who had been initially hesitant.

Environmental Culture

Other departments may resist working within a collaborative model because open communication means sharing information. There are always departments where managers prefer to withhold information because they mistakenly believe that their power is directly proportional to the secrets of their operation. They believe they have better control if certain operations are unknown.

Improvement Strategies

Set an example by sharing information that is traditionally viewed as secretive. I chose to give the full-time nursing faculty a copy of their departmental budget, exclusive of staff salaries. I asked them for suggestions for expenditures and solicited their help in writing justifications for additional monies. When faculty had access to information and were asked to participate in decision making, they felt empowered and supportive of the department.

Collective Bargaining Unit

Some faculty members were advised by the union to be nonsupportive of any team processes that involved shared power. Unions need to maintain an adversarial image with administration for survival.

Improvement Strategies

Be honest and supportive of faculty, eliminate an adversarial relationship and use data to support decisions. Make a conscious commitment to be a leader. This is very hard because most of us are caught in a management paradigm.

SUGGESTED LEADERSHIP STRATEGIES

Some leadership strategies that I have used to support shared power include:

- Understand the needs, goals, and capabilities of individuals in your organization.
- Recognize that it is your job to help your staff be the best they can be.
- Choose team leaders who crave responsibilities, take risks, and are decisive.
- Build strong alliances. A house divided against itself cannot stand.
- Be a strong, supportive leader. Your organization will take on the personality of its top management.
- Seek first to understand!

- Do not allow yourself the luxury of negative decision making.
- Delegate, don't DUMP!

POWER BOOSTERS

Activities that you can do to boost someone's self-esteem and empower them to be the best they can be are "Power Boosters," for example:

- Catch someone doing something right and praise them.
- Write someone a letter of commendation and copy it to their personnel file and to the person to whom they report.
- Drive out fear!
- Use data-driven decision making to avoid acting on assumptions.

A PERSONAL CODE OF LEADERSHIP

I would like to share my personal code of leadership with all of you (see Figure 2). It has helped me lead others to work toward their potential. An important perspective to remember is: Once you reach the top, then turn around, reach down and help the person behind you up to the top. Remember, if at all possible: *Leave a legacy of leadership.*

Figure 2.   A Personal Code of Leadership

I WILL:
- SEEK FIRST TO UNDERSTAND.
- HELP EACH PERSON TO BE THE BEST THAT HE/SHE CAN BE.
- CREATE AN ENVIRONMENT WHERE PEOPLE CAN BE AUTONOMOUS AND RESPONSIBLE.
- SHARE DECISION MAKING.
- ENCOURAGE, RECOGNIZE AND REWARD THOSE WHO TAKE OWNERSHIP OF THEIR DESTINIES.
- BE DECISIVE AND CONSISTENT.
- AVOID NEGATIVITY.
- NEITHER PRACTICE NOR ENTERTAIN WHINING.

PART III

Faculty Change: New Opportunities to Embrace Ambiguity

9

Creating an Environment for Faculty Change: How One Faculty Member Joined the Curriculum Revolution and Lived to Tell about It

Jeanette Bernhardt
Marie Guynn

I want to tell you about a journey: a journey that began for each of us at different times and different places. I can only tell you my personal beginning and how the journey progressed from my perspective. There are other stories in this publication by some of my colleagues: Carol Wilson, Carolyn Hickox, and Karen Rankin. Their stories are somewhat different.

Several years ago, Pat Conroy, a southern author, was the speaker at a convocation at West Georgia College. In his remarks that day, he celebrated the best of the South. He also spoke of teaching, the role of teacher and the role of learner. He reminded the audience of the story of Zorba the Greek and the young man who begged Zorba to teach him to dance. In his final remarks, he urged those of us in the audience to teach our students all the good things about the South—and to teach them to dance. I didn't know it at the time but this speech was a paradigm experience for me. Actually, I had to go back to school to know what a paradigm experience was; then I could name it!

Conroy's remarks really hit home with me because I really did not think that our students were learning to dance; that is, the process of learning didn't appear to be much fun. In fact, nursing education, as I knew it, appeared to be stressful, punitive, and at times, downright painful. I filed those thoughts away, but they became the tip of a huge iceberg. I now believe that we are beginning to teach our students to dance.

During the academic year 1988–89, the faculty began what was to become a long journey as we pondered several questions about the future of our program. One predominant question we asked was this: Do we keep the ASN program and the RN to BSN program or should we have a generic BSN or what? We tried to decide what the future of nursing would be and what skills and attitudes our graduates would need for the future.

Individually and collectively, the following observations were made:

1. Hospitalized patients were sicker and hospital stays were shorter, thus necessitating that nurses possess increased technical, problem-solving, and teaching skills.
2. New graduates were not getting the support they needed in the workplace to become confident practitioners.
3. Graduates felt frustrated in their efforts to effect change, were frequently changing jobs, or were adopting the attitudes and practices of their co-workers that they had once criticized and had difficulty understanding.
4. Our students were brighter and more enthusiastic upon entering nursing school but were burned out and less enthusiastic about both nursing and education by graduation.
5. Faculty were packing more and more information into class and students were complaining about information overload. We had what I call the *Hefty Bag concept* about curriculum.
6. We were committed to facilitating better articulation between the ASN and RN-BSN programs.

During fall 1989 quarter, as the curriculum committee began the work of defining a new philosophy, individual faculty began to complete a series of questions. For several Mondays, questions appeared in faculty mailboxes with strict instructions to return them by Thursday. The questions were:

- What is nursing?
- What are characteristics of the ideal graduate? Employee? New nurse?

- What is essential for nurses to know versus what is nice to know?

The curriculum committee compiled all the answers and begin to write the framework of a new philosophy. At the end of fall quarter that year, a faculty retreat was planned. We told the person making the arrangements to be frugal. She succeeded in securing a cabin in a state park in Alabama that slept eight for $64/night. We left early one morning with plans to return after lunch the next day. The cabin did indeed sleep eight people in an assortment of bunkbeds, double beds, and whatever. The bathroom was an architectural afterthought. The cabin had one large room which served as kitchen, living room, and bedroom. One other room, a screened porch, had more beds. But we had a good time, the restaurant was very nice, and of course, we took enough snacks to feed a small army. At the end of the retreat, our vision was still a little fuzzy, but definitely beginning to take shape.

Our next step was to meet with clinical advisory groups and students. We did this in December 1990. After these meetings, numerous conversations, and a second retreat—this time much more upscale—we listed the following characteristics as those we wanted to see in our graduates:

1. To be caring—able to care for self, patients, peers (fellow students and co-workers), and their world (to be good citizens).
2. To be scholarly individuals—to know how to think and make decisions, how to seek and evaluate information, how to weigh options and how to convince others of the need for change.
3. To recognize the influence of mind, body, and spirit on well-being and how to foster this positive relationship in themselves and others.

The acceptance of these assumptions challenged us to consider the nature of the nursing program at West Georgia College. If we wanted to foster these attitudes in our students, we had to make changes in the program and in our teaching methodologies. This brings me to a very important point: If we want to change nursing as we know it or at least improve nursing care substantially, we must change the way we teach nursing! During the time we were holding retreats and meetings and developing a new philosophy, other things were changing and affecting the way we viewed curriculum, students, the world, and ourselves. One predominant factor was the workload issue. Faculty in the nursing department were expected to be as scholarly as other faculty; that is, to write, present, and publish. Time became even more precious as one more task was added to an already crowded schedule. The faculty begin to consider another question: What can we give up? What are we doing that can be done differently or perhaps not at all? We began to let go of some of the traditional tasks of nursing faculty. Students were allowed to check off each other in lab and to make their own clinical assignments. We even let them write their own clinical evaluations.

At about the same time, one of our students said to us, "You know, nursing students don't have to look for anything. You tell them exactly what they need to know and usually provide most of the information." She also commented that this was not the way she was treated in other courses, when faculty expected students to be able to locate information other than what was furnished in class.

Another factor which became significant was the use of more part-time faculty. One faculty member commented to me that, believe it or not, sharing the load with more people was really more time consuming. Through all of this I sensed a quiet uneasiness among the faculty. There had to be a better way to do things.

As a result, the faculty began a definite shift in world views. We shifted from making sure that no student who took boards would fail to making sure that all students who took boards had a good chance of passing. That is a very subtle but a very significant change.

The faculty also moved from being failure-oriented to being success-oriented. And possibly most significantly, the faculty moved from knowing what students needed to know to knowing that students needed to know how to learn; from being controllers of learning to facilitators of learning. And, last, we wanted students to know the joy of learning!

When the philosophy was written, the objectives identified, and the assumptions articulated, the following changes were made in the program of learning:

1. The number of credit hours for each nursing course was decreased, making it feasible for one or two people to teach a single course rather than larger teaching teams. We basically abandoned the team teaching concept.

2. The total number of hours in the ASN program was reduced from 51 quarter hours to 45 and in the RN-BSN program from 41 to 38 to facilitate articulation between the two programs and to be competitive with generic BSN programs.

3. The same number of actual clinical hours was maintained by including a heavy practicum (24 hours/week) in the last quarter.

4. The faculty critically examined what was essential content versus what was nice to know. This continues to be an on-going debate as individual faculty members consider their own beloved content.

5. Several sections of each class were scheduled to accommodate smaller classes of 20 to 25 students rather than larger classes of 40 to 50. Several sections of clinical laboratory experience were also scheduled which better utilized clinical space and time. With this plan, most faculty have at least one day without class or clinical, which allows time to write and prepare presentations.

6. Skills classes were separated from theory classes. When we met with clinical agency representatives, their biggest concern was technical competence. Students were also concerned about competence, so time was set aside to focus on the technical skills of nursing.

7. In the classroom, every effort was made to maintain an egalitarian atmosphere—all are learners and all are teachers. We appreciate what each person can contribute; the teacher is the facilitator of learning rather than the giver of information. Desks in the classroom are usually arranged in a circle.

8. Classroom activities became reality-based and participatory. There was less lecture, more discussion, and group work as students learned to become critical thinkers. Case studies and common clinical problems became the basis of classroom discussions.

9. The cornerstones of the curriculum—caring, critical thinking, and holism—became the foci of classroom and clinical activities. Caring groups, groups of faculty and students, were implemented for the express purpose of intentionally caring for self and others. Activities were planned to assist students to enhance their own wellness and to support an integration of

mind-body-spirit in patients and in themselves. Learning strategies to encourage critical thinking were intentionally included.

So, what data do we have that this is working? For one thing, attrition is low. In fact, for the past three years, attrition has been less than 10 percent due to failure in nursing.

Second, ASN students are moving directly into the RN-BSN program. Last year, 25 percent of the graduating class and this year approximately 37 percent of the graduating class continued enrollment in the RN-BSN program. This is a big change from approximately 5 percent continuing in the RN-BSN program.

Third, while students from this curriculum won't take NCLEX until the summer of 1994, faculty have used essentially the same classroom tests and students continue to do well.

Additionally, there is some hard data that this approach may be working. A colleague who was completing a dissertation about students' coping skills involved our students in her research (Rollant, 1993). Using a coping skills inventory as a pre- and post-test, this colleague used three groups of associate degree students. Our students, who were involved in specific learning activities related to stress, were better able to recognize stress and do something to reduce it than students who took the coping test with no feedback and those who took the coping test with feedback.

There are some observations we have made about our students. Students appear to be more enthusiastic about nursing. Students generally appear to be more confident. Confident students make good learners. Because students are responsible for their own actions, faculty don't have to play the heavy so often.

Publications in the department have increased exponentially, from three in 1991, to six in 1992, and to nine in 1993. Three RN-BSN students have publications. So far this year, a total of six faculty members have been involved in national and/or regional presentations and six faculty members have written manuscripts that have been accepted for publication.

Has the journey been easy? No. Has the pain been worth it? Yes. If you grow, you must experience a little pain. If you choose to dream, you have to be willing to have a few nightmares. Did the faculty have some monumental arguments? You bet.

For some years, I have believed that the best nursing faculty in the world is composed of two very special kinds of individuals.

Some individuals need to be dreamers. They really do live in an ivory tower. Questions frequently asked by the dreamers are "What if . . . ?" and "Why don't we do . . . ?" The other individuals need to be realists. Their feet are firmly planted on the ground. Their comments frequently are "Get real. . . ." and "Because. . . ." If you are fortunate to have these individuals, and if the dreamers and the realists will listen to each other, your journey will not only be successful, but also it will be fun!

Em Bevis, in her book, *Toward a Caring Curriculum,* gave us this advice, "So here we are with a dream to build, hopes to fulfill, visions to realize, and a future to construct" (1989, p. 64). I invite you to join us in this journey. Dare to dream dreams about nursing education; help us construct a new vision for nursing education!

REFERENCES

Bevis, E.O., & Watson, J. (1989). *Toward a caring curriculum: A new pedagogy for nursing.* New York: National League for Nursing Press.

Rollant, P.D. (1993). A comparison of effects of interventions upon stress coping resources of beginning associate degree nursing students. Georgia State University.

10

Caring Groups: An Experiential Teaching/Learning Strategy

Carol Wilson
Carolyn Hickox

*C*aring interactions among students and faculty increase caring behaviors in both groups. This statement reflects the philosophy of
the Department of Nursing at West Georgia College. The faculty
shares the belief of others (Nelms, Jones, & Gray, 1993) that caring
can be taught. It is a way of being that is intentionally brought to
awareness and role modeled for students. Students and faculty are
given an opportunity to practice caring behaviors in a safe environment that may increase the practice of caring behaviors in future
nursing practice. The use of caring groups in nursing education is
an experiential teaching/learning strategy that teaches participants
to care for themselves, others, and their environment.

The nursing faculty at West Georgia College became aware of the
need to teach caring as the central core of nursing in a variety of
ways. Two of our faculty members participated in caring courses and
caring groups as a part of the coursework for the PhD in nursing at
Georgia State University in Atlanta, Georgia. These faculty members
verbalized a very positive experience and expressed a desire to provide a similar experience for students. One faculty member became
involved in the American Holistic Nurses Association and participated
in activities with this group. Faculty members also attended national
conferences on caring in nursing education, read publications related
to caring and the curriculum revolution published by the National
League for Nursing, and began to learn about the curriculum revolution with an emphasis on caring and transformative student-teacher

relationships. Excitement was generated as we began to read and dialogue about the work of Em Bevis (1988), Bevis and Murray (1990), Pat Moccia (1990), Jean Watson (1989), Nancy Diekelman (1991), and other significant contributors to the curriculum revolution. The call for a true revolution in nursing education seemed to be a call we wanted to follow.

The need for teaching nursing students how to care for themselves as well as each other was realized. The desired outcome of teaching caring and encouraging students to learn to care for self and others has increased caring behaviors in nursing practice. Critics of the curriculum revolution have said that as nurses we know how to care, since caring is a natural process, and there is no need to worry about explicitly incorporating this concept into nursing education programs. The faculty and students at West Georgia College had observed, however, that nurses in practice do not practice caring behaviors with themselves or each other. The nursing faculty at West Georgia College believes, and the curriculum revolution supports, that providing students an opportunity to learn and practice caring will translate into caring behaviors related to patients, co-workers, families, friends, and strangers.

As the faculty at West Georgia College began to embrace the tenants of the curriculum revolution, we experienced a paradigm shift. Through reading, studying, and talking with each other, we realized that a conscious focus on caring behaviors felt right for us. Our student-teacher relationship was gradually transformed to a more collegial one that resembles a partnership in the learning process. While it is acknowledged that the power differential still exists (since the teacher does hold power in terms of the grading and evaluation process), efforts have been made to create a context in which the student is more of a participant in the learning process. The idea is to decrease the power differential as much as possible.

Caring groups were initiated as one teaching/learning strategy designed to implement a curriculum based on caring. It is the belief of the faculty at West Georgia College that participation in caring groups, during which caring interactions among group members occur, encourages students and faculty to be caring individuals.

ESTABLISHING THE GROUPS

Caring groups have been established as a strategy to provide activities that will enable the participants to learn how to care for themselves, for others, and for their environment. The overall purposes of this activity are to provide a way for students and faculty to give and receive care, to develop self-awareness and empowerment, and most of all, to recognize that care of self precedes caring for others.

Caring groups are organized during the first quarter of the associate degree nursing program. Each group includes 10 to 12 students and a faculty facilitator. Students are randomly assigned to a caring group based on the clinical group for which they register the first quarter. This initial group and faculty facilitator remain together as a caring group throughout the entire nursing program. Although it has been suggested that groups be reorganized for the second year, students have elected to remain with the same group throughout the program. Many students commented that the primary reason for wanting to keep the groups the same was related to the amount of time it takes to establish support and trust within the group, which is essential for the group to progress.

Each caring group meets from four to six hours a quarter. Students are given clinical credit for the time spent in the caring group. Clinical time for participation is given because faculty believe that it is very valuable time with the students; time that is as important as any other clinical experience in which students participate.

Caring groups provide an opportunity for students to share their concerns and feelings in a safe environment. Nursing students have special concerns that other students on campus do not have. Faculty believe it is important to have some type of support among the students themselves. Initial meetings focus on establishing group trust and cohesiveness. In any group, this is necessary to progress in becoming comfortable sharing problems and concerns.

Group Goals

In addition to activities that will help establish group trust, each group establishes group goals during the initial meetings of the group. These include: *learning to care for self and others and identifying caring and noncaring behaviors* observed in group members, peers, and nurses in various clinical settings. These behaviors are discussed during caring group meetings. Although very idealistic at this point in their nursing education, students are skilled at perceiving caring and noncaring behaviors in nurses as well as others. The group provides the opportunity to discuss these various behaviors and receive feedback on perceptions.

Problem solving takes place depending on what needs arise in the group. *Having fun* is one of the major stress reduction techniques used. Each group finds its own way of fulfilling this need.

Learning to ask for help is difficult for some people. Faculty try to assist students in understanding the need to ask for assistance when needed.

Affirming each other provides support and encouragement for each group member. Telling another what one likes about him or her, what is good about him or her, and de-emphasizing the negative is a good way to reinforce self-esteem and awareness of strengths.

Personal Goals

Some students set personal goals that they wish to work on individually. These may include trying not to monopolize the group; sharing time with other group members so that everybody has a chance to talk if desired; asking for support when needed; becoming more assertive in giving and receiving feedback; and supporting other group members when needed. It is important for all the members to understand that sometimes you give and sometimes you receive.

Each individual group functions and progresses differently depending on the composition of the group and the wishes and desires of the group. Groups tend to progress at different rates as they work on different tasks. What takes place in each group is confidential. The faculty facilitator tends to be the leader of the group initially, although at times students may take on the leadership role. Faculty believe this is a good way to learn both group process as well as the responsibilities of being a leader. In addition, the philosophy of the faculty is to view the student in a more collegial manner. This helps students understand that faculty really do believe students and faculty are of equal importance in the teaching-learning process.

GROUP GUIDELINES

It is important during the initial establishment of the group that students and faculty facilitator establish some rules regarding participation and attendance. These may be written rules in the form of a contract or they can be verbal rules. Of utmost importance is the need for maintaining confidentiality. This not only promotes a safe environment to share feelings, but also reinforces the concept of confidentiality when dealing with patients. Many times group members will share things that they feel comfortable sharing because of the confidentiality of the group—things that might go unsaid otherwise.

Each group member, and this includes the faculty facilitator, needs to listen attentively and give feedback to other group members. The faculty facilitator does no more talking than any other group member in order that students will become more comfortable participating in the group. It is of importance to note that faculty at times share things that they might not have been comfortable sharing with students in the past.

Demonstrating a respectful attitude toward other group members is required. Maintaining a nonjudgmental and accepting attitude is critical, as nursing students, as well as the patient population, become increasingly diverse. The caring group has given students the opportunity to become more tolerant of the behavior of others and much less judgmental in accepting others, as well as patients, who might have different value systems, religions, and sociocultural backgrounds.

Being honest, talking, and sharing feelings with other group members is expected of each group member. Allowing and encouraging others to talk is promoted. When this expectation is established in the beginning, each group member knows everybody can have their own time when needed. The faculty facilitator no longer has to provide the impetus to encourage a group member to participate. As the group progresses, it is interesting to observe students encouraging other students to participate.

STRATEGIES AND ACTIVITIES

The initial meeting of the caring group involves participation in a *Ropes Course*. This is an outdoor group activity that promotes problem solving, group support, and trust building. The activity lasts eight hours and clinical time is used for this. The *Ropes Course* has been very productive in the establishment of the groups as faculty and students all feel it is a wonderful way to build group cohesiveness. The physical activities and games are designed to meet the goals of the activity.

Group discussion is used during every meeting. The focus of the discussion depends on individual group needs. Most groups will begin a group meeting with what is termed a check in such as, "Well, how are you doing?", "How's everybody been since our last meeting?", or "Is there anything special we need to talk about?" The discussion will usually move forward from this point. Students observe in several different types of nursing and health care settings during the first quarter. Much time is spent in discussing perceptions of caring and noncaring behaviors observed during these experiences. These discussions increase students' awareness of the importance of caring, which is a major focus of the philosophy at West Georgia College.

At times, feelings and concerns are shared through group discussion. At other times, problem solving may occur. Sometimes, self-disclosure occurs during group discussion. A student may need somebody to talk to and is willing to share that with the group. Many nursing students are married and have families, must work, or have other things that place demands on their time. Classroom concerns or personal concerns regarding issues at home and their effects on school may be discussed.

Affirmation exercises are used to build self-confidence. Several card and board games are available that help affirm positive qualities. An example of an affirmation exercise is to ask each group member to identify positive attributes and strengths in other group members.

Relaxation and stress reduction techniques are taught, demonstrated, and practiced during caring group meetings. Faculty use tapes, exercises, and music to teach students visualization and relaxation. Students continue to use these techniques throughout the program. A coping skills inventory is administered to students that gives feedback regarding strengths. Humor is a wonderful way to reduce stress. Relaxation can occur through telling jokes, sharing funny stories, and just having a good time. Parties and eating are used to promote relaxation and to get away from the stress of school. Baby and wedding showers are sometimes the modus operandi. Many students feel if you have not eaten at a caring group meeting it does not count, so someone usually brings food. One caring group decided to go out for breakfast and then went to a costume shop where they tried on costumes and took photos.

Games are used not only for affirmation exercises but also to have fun, promote self-disclosure, develop more assertive behaviors, and get to know one another better. One faculty had each group member name something that is liked about self and something each would like to work on—not something negative or bad, but something to improve on. Another activity is to have each group member complete the following three sentences:

I feel _____.
I need _____.
I want _____.

Each group member completes these sentences and comments on them. An additional activity is to have each group member make three statements about self, only one of which is true. The other group members must identify the true statement. One group brought baby pictures to the faculty facilitator. The facilitator organized the photos on a display board and at the next meeting members had to identify each other from the pictures.

Assertiveness practice can occur in a safe, nonthreatening environment during caring group meetings. Group members may have some conflicts among themselves or with others. The caring group provides a medium whereby members are aware of the need to be assertive, that is, constructive in feedback, rather than hurtful and are able to practice this behavior and resolve conflicts knowing they will be supported by other group members. In one instance, two group members who became confrontive were supported by the rest of the group in resolving the conflict. Following the experience, group members verbalized positive feelings about the outcome.

If a group member feels that caring group is not beneficial, for whatever reason, dialogue journaling can be offered as an alternative to participation in caring group. The student is asked to write comments about experiences when caring or noncaring occurs; how they feel or how they might have acted differently; or whatever they feel a need to discuss. In this instance, the faculty facilitator provides ongoing feedback to the student in the form of a confidential conversation. Some students have participated in this alternative activity. Some have later rejoined the group as a participating member.

There are several other alternatives to participation in caring group that can be offered to those students that do not find caring group to be beneficial or for some reason do not feel comfortable sharing things in a group. One alternative considered was having students read an article on caring and write a synopsis of the article when a caring group meeting is missed. However, students felt this to be a nonconstructive and punitive measure, so this option was discarded. Students have suggested that for those students who chose to not participate in caring group or do not want to journal, an option of volunteering time in a community project of some sort, such as a food kitchen, hospice, or other community service project might be appropriate.

During their final quarter, students participate in an extensive preceptorship. Consequently, it is extremely difficult to arrange meeting times for caring groups. As an alternative, the group meets at the beginning of the quarter and plans a mutually satisfactory date to meet at the end of this final quarter in the program. Throughout the quarter, as each student assimilates and processes the various clinical experiences that occur in practice, they are asked to write short anecdotal stories that reflect instances of caring in themselves as well as others. At the end of the quarter, they are asked to share these stories of caring during the last caring group meeting. During this final meeting, when closure of the group is occurring, students reflect on their growth and progress throughout the program as well as how they as individuals have learned to care. The anecdotal stories reinforce this.

INFORMAL SURVEY RESULTS

During the spring quarter 1993, an informal survey was done at West Georgia College to collect data on the experience of caring groups from student and faculty perspectives. A review of the literature related to caring in nursing education supported the idea of caring groups (Beck, 1992; Hover-Kramer, 1989; Hughes, 1992, 1993; Miller, Haber, & Byrne, 1990; Slevin & Harter, 1987). No data was available, however, that documented the outcome of activities such as caring groups.

The results of the informal survey indicate that participation in caring groups is generally a positive experience for students and faculty. The students were asked to respond to the question, "How do you feel participation in caring group has changed your relationship with your classmates?" Many students stated they felt it was a good way of getting to know each other on a personal and meaningful level. Participation in caring group was seen as an opportunity to give and receive support in times of crisis. Students recognized the need to learn how to care for themselves before they could care for others. This recognition of the need to learn to care for self before it is possible to care for others was an important goal of the faculty for the caring groups. The realization that caring is an attitude as well as an action was expressed. The caring group meetings were perceived as a time to share interests other than studies as well as common concerns.

One of the themes reflected in the caring group survey was related to sharing. Statements written in support of the caring groups indicated that we share common problems. Students felt it was helpful to find out that other people in the classroom experienced similar kinds of problems and concerns. A second theme expressed by caring group participants in the survey was related to togetherness. With a caring group, students have a support system and truly get to know each other well.

Students and faculty were asked about the perceptions of the effect of participation in caring group on relationships with patients. Students' comments included, "I am more aware of the importance of caring as the main component in helping patients" and "I have developed more empathy toward patients." Patients were perceived more holistically as having a need to talk about things not directly related to illness. Carol Lindeman (1994) supports the idea that nursing education needs to be doing more than teaching students to apply scientific principles to illnesses. Dr. Lindeman indicated that students need to be taught to look at patients holistically. Quite often when we interact with a patient to provide physical care, which often involves many technical skills, we are not aware of what the patient perceives to be the most important concern. Therefore, we need to teach students to look at patients more holistically.

Students were asked to respond to ways in which they may have changed as a result of participation in caring group. The theme that emerged from this question was feeling cared for as a precursor to caring for others. One student stated, "I show more caring because I feel more cared for." Another student indicated, "Knowing others care for me makes me care more for others."

The response of faculty to this same question indicated a perception of becoming more sensitive to their own and others caring interactions with patients as well as being more aware of modeling caring behaviors. Faculty indicated a perception of raised consciousness when interacting with a patient under a student's observation. Faculty indicated the belief that students learn caring as caring behaviors are role modeled for them.

Students were asked to respond to questions about faculty. Faculty were perceived as supportive, caring, less intimidating, and "a friend I can turn to for advice." A common theme in the survey was related to students' realization that faculty are human too and have feelings. In traditional nursing education programs the emphasis was on distance in relationships with students in order to maintain objectivity. Many of us would become involved in what we considered an ethical dilemma when we found ourselves becoming too friendly with our students. One of the major concepts of the curriculum revolution focuses on a redefinition of the student-teacher relationship (National League for Nursing, 1990). As our faculty embraced the tenets of the curriculum revolution we altered our way-of-being with our students. The student-teacher relationship is now seen as one of collegiality and partnership. Evidence of our success in these efforts was indicated in the survey when students responded that they see us as equal rather than superior.

Students were asked about the impact, if any, which participation in caring group had made in relationships with family and friends. A common theme related to the ability to express feelings in the supportive environment of a caring group. Some students indicated that this made it easier to express feelings with family and friends. Students who indicated they did not have supportive family environments felt the caring group provided the needed support.

In terms of caring relationships with strangers, students reported they felt they were more open and accepting of others. The importance of being less judgmental and of avoiding assumptions based on first impressions was expressed. This is a concept which receives considerable focus in the caring groups based on a critical thinking perspective. Activities related to this include values clarification exercises.

The results of the survey indicated that the experience of participation in caring groups is generally a positive one for both students and faculty. The faculty at West Georgia College is committed to continuing the caring groups. A qualitative research study is currently being conducted for two years with the first group of students to graduate following participation in caring groups. The results of this study will hopefully provide data to support the continuation of the caring groups.

THE BURDEN OF CARING

We acknowledge that there is another side to the experience of caring groups, or the *burden of caring*. The caring group creates a context in which self-disclosure of a student may occur. This self-disclosure may reveal personal information creating a situation uncomfortable for the faculty member because it goes beyond the purpose of the caring group. The student may disclose a problem that needs intervention beyond the qualifications of the nursing faculty. To be prepared for such situations, the caring group faculty facilitator must be aware of resources available to assist the student in any way that might be needed. The West Georgia College counseling center has been helpful in responding to our requests for assistance for students.

Faculty have experienced situations in which students have disclosed personal information about themselves that faculty perceived as needing immediate intervention. Appointments were made and students were accompanied to the counseling center. Other less serious situations have resulted in faculty recommending a student seek counseling. The concept of self-disclosure raises questions related to differentiating between the faculty's role as facilitator of a support group and the role of counselor. For example, if a student discloses a problem with drugs or alcohol, what is done with this information? Ideally, there are policies in place supporting the student to seek treatment.

Another burden for the faculty participating in caring groups is the time commitment. A caring support group may include 10 or 12 students. The nature of the group supports the development of trusting relationships among group members. A student may feel uncomfortable disclosing information in a group setting, yet may come to the faculty facilitator individually. The time commitment for providing individual support may go well beyond the time allotted within the faculty's teaching assignment for caring groups.

Faculty members indicated an increased awareness, as we have participated in caring groups with students, of the need to be more supportive of each other. Some days a faculty member may be really busy and stressed. They may find themselves wondering how much more caring they have left to give. Faculty need to learn how to care for themselves as well. A faculty caring group is needed. However, a formal caring group for faculty is something we have not yet implemented at West Georgia College, although we plan to do so in the future. Our faculty is small and very cohesive. We often have informal meetings in which we share problems and concerns and provide support for each other. We recognize, however, this would be more difficult with a larger faculty.

CONCLUSION

The faculty at West Georgia College believe that caring is a way of being and is essential to nursing. If nursing students are to value and practice caring, they must have the opportunity to experience and learn about caring. It is this opportunity that we are trying to provide for our students.

REFERENCES

Beck, C. (1992). Caring among nursing students. *Nurse Educator. 17*(6), 22–27.

Bevis, E. O. (1988). New directions for a new age. In *Curriculum revolution: Mandate for change.* (pp. 27–51). New York: National League for Nursing Press.

Bevis, E. O., & Murray, J. (1990). The essence of the curriculum revolution: Emancipatory teaching. *Journal of Nursing Education. 29*(7), 326–331.

Diekelman, N. (1991). The emancipatory power of the narrative. In *Curriculum revolution: Community building and activism.* (pp. 41–62). New York: National League for Nursing Press.

Hover-Kramer, D. (1989). Creating a context for self-healing: The transpersonal perspective. *Holistic Nursing Practice. 3*(3), 27–34.

Hughes, L. (1992). Faculty-student interactions and the student perceived climate for caring. *Advances in Nursing Science. 4*(3), 60–71.

Hughes, L. (1993). Peer group interactions and the student perceived climate for caring. *Journal of Nursing Education. 32*(2), 78–83.

Lindeman, C. (1994). The web of inclusion: Faculty helping faculty. National League for Nursing, Council of Associate Degree Programs. Crystal City, Virginia, April 5, 1994.

Miller, B., Haber, J., & Byrne, M. (1990). The experience of caring in the teaching learning process of nursing education: Student and teacher perspectives. In M. Leininger & J. Watson, (Eds.), *The caring imperative in nursing education.* New York: National League for Nursing Press.

Moccia, P. (1990). No sire, it's a revolution. *Journal of Nursing Education. 29*(7), 27–29.

Nelms, T., Jones, J., & Gray, P. (1993). Role modeling: A method for teaching caring in nursing education. *Journal of Nursing Education. 32*(1), 18–22.

National League for Nursing. (1990). *Curriculum revolution: Redefining the student-teacher relationship.* New York: National League for Nursing Press.

Watson, J. (1989). Transformative thinking and a caring curriculum. In *Toward a caring curriculum: A new pedagogy for nursing.* New York: National League for Nursing Press.

11

Bridging the Gap in Generational Understanding: Shared Learning Between the Well-Elderly Client and Nursing Students

Karen L. Rankin

*A*n innovative way to focus on geriatric concepts, integrated into the Psych-Mental Health curriculum, can be accomplished through the use of a *Well-Elderly Interview*. The focus of the activity is to help the student gain experience in therapeutic communication through an in-depth understanding and insight into the joys and problems of aging.

McBride and Burgener (1994) note that early in the twenty-first century, 20 percent of the population will be over 65 and persons over 85 will triple within 50 years. Predicted changes in the role of nursing, both present and future, indicate the need for an accelerated approach to health care focused in the community setting (Ebersole, 1991). Understanding the societal parameters associated with aging encourages critical thinking in problem solving. This is especially important in the planning and implementation of care of the elderly because of the complexity of the social, economic, physical, and psychologic presentation of needs. The student, together with the client, can validate and evaluate what helps and hinders their participation in daily activities and routines.

The student contracts with an individual over the age of 68 and living independently in the community to meet for six one (1) to two (2) hour, in-depth interviews. The sessions focus on life history, developmental tasks, health history and assessment, grief and loss, nutrition, and personal and environmental safety.

The interview helps to form a positive outlook on aging as a result of the communicative bond between the student and the elderly individual. The student gains a clearer understanding of the normal physiological and psychosocial changes occurring with advancing chronological age. Emphasis is placed on relating learned developmental theory with observed or verbalized content from the client. A holistic focus guides the interview process in assessing and understanding the information shared by the older adult.

Through increased awareness of the lived experiences associated with aging, the student and client develop mutual respect and trust. This results in an open dialogue enabling understanding of the impact of aging on daily living.

Together, they explore how those with chronic conditions can live very productive, healthy, fulfilling lives despite their limitations. The image of the elderly person as an infirm and helpless individual is diminished by listening to the descriptions of their childhood and adult life experiences and accomplishments. Frequently, the student recognizes that the hopes and dreams of the elderly directly reflect their own aspirations in life.

Emphasis is placed on knowing and caring for self to facilitate a nonjudgmental, positive regard for the client's journey through the older adult years. As part of the caring approach, needed changes in the health care system are also explored.

Problem solving is used to meet identified psychosocial and physiological needs of the elderly. Hegner and Caldwell (1991) state the needs of the elderly are similar to the basic needs of all age groups. The need for love and affection and adequate resources for food and shelter are shared requirements. The students focus on ways to facilitate wellness behaviors and outcomes in the aging population. Available resources to meet the health care needs of the elderly, at a local and federal level, are analyzed for accessibility, feasibility, and effectiveness. Analysis of issues impacting on the well elderly serves as the groundwork for planning and intervening with the acutely ill elderly person in the hospital setting.

Solutions to problematic issues, identified by the client in the interviews, are generated by exchange of ideas among the students. These are shared with the elderly client for validation of the plan's usefulness to their specific needs.

By critically analyzing the various aspects of aging, a forum is created whereby students can discuss ways to plan and problem solve to meet the health and societal needs of the present and future elderly population. Malek (1986), in discussing teaching methods to promote critical thinking, believed success in teaching critical thinking involved pacing and sequential learning built on a sound knowledge base. The theoretical content on aging is directly related to the student's experiential analysis of the elder interview.

In addition to the interviews, the student records personal thoughts and feelings in a daily journal to encourage self-awareness of the nurse's role, therapeutic communication, and the interpretation of verbal dialogue with the client. The journal is shared with a faculty member and serves as a vehicle for reciprocal exchange of ideas, feelings, and positive feedback between the faculty and student. This process nourishes the student's sense of self-worth and encourages trust in others through the acknowledgment of their ideas. Another function of the journal process is identifying the underlying messages that occur in interpersonal communication.

Using principles of critical thinking, group seminars are planned to discuss how the activity has influenced the student's thinking toward aging and the older adult. Students are encouraged to internalize and analyze the data from the interviews. In the seminar setting and through the journal writing, personal values and attitudes are clarified in a caring and trusting atmosphere. This helps the student to analyze how their predetermined assumptions and opinions influence interactions with others.

Through acknowledging the elderly's role in the community and their contributions to society in general, the student gains a realization of the importance of supporting each person's effort in retaining the freedom to choose in all facets of daily living. Understanding the dynamics of aging, within the societal context, encourages student awareness of the need to create their own personal plan for aging in regard to community resources and access to health care.

The student's evaluation of the activity, both written and verbal, is positive and indicates a view of the older individual as part of his or her world. By acknowledging the contributions to society by the elderly, the student is better able to support the older patient in retaining control over treatment decisions when faced with the limitations of an acute or chronic illness.

By gaining insight into their thinking regarding aspects of aging, the student is able to evaluate issues related to societal norms in relation to the growing elderly population. To quote a student, "I thought that all old people did was sit in a chair all day long doing nothing, but instead I found they strive to occupy their time constructively and plan and dream about their future happiness just like me!"

REFERENCES

Burke, M., & Sherman, S. (Eds.). (1993). *Ways of knowing and caring for older adults.* New York: National League for Nursing Press.

Council of Associate Degree Programs. (1992). *Educational outcomes of associate degree programs: Roles and competencies.* New York: National League for Nursing Press.

Ebersole, P. (1990). The future of gerontic nursing. *Imprint/NSNA, 37*(4), 59–61.

Hegner, B., & Caldwell, E. (1991). *Geriatrics: A study of maturity.* (5th ed.). Albany: Delmar.

McBride, A., & Burgener, S. (1994). Strategies to implement geropsychiatric nursing curricula content. *Journal of Psychosocial Nursing, 32*(4), 13–18.

Malek, C. (1986). A Model for teaching critical thinking. *Nurse Educator, 11*:20–23.

Winnick, Hull, & Delp. (1991). Honoring elders: Empowering caregivers. *Advancing Clinical Care,* 8–10.

12

A Study of Student Retention in Associate Degree Nursing Programs as Perceived by Their Directors

Linda L. Hunt

*R*etaining qualified students is an evergrowing challenge for nursing educators. Fewer students are entering and completing nursing programs than in past years (Rosenfeld, 1988). It is important that college environments enhance student satisfaction and success in an attempt to decrease the number of qualified students who drop out of programs.

Rosenfeld (1988) reported a National League for Nursing study on retention rates in nursing programs during 1985–86. The retention rate for associate degree nursing programs was in the low 80 percent range: 83.6 percent for public and 81.8 percent for private institutions. However, in the same study 50 percent of all directors of nursing programs reported having difficulty retaining students.

Meissner (1986) wrote that nurses are "eating their young" by setting unrealistic expectations not only for the new graduate but also for the nursing student. "If nurses really want to see nursing achieve professional status, each of us—educators, administrators, and practitioners—must reexamine our interactions with novice nurses" (Meissner, 1986, p. 53). Although she did not write specifically about retention of nursing students, she associated this attitude with failure of nursing students to thrive.

According to Cope (1987), persistence in college results from more than individual characteristics of students; it is also a result of the characteristics of the college or university. Although research on college characteristics does not provide firm guidelines;

the research regarding integrating the individual student within the social and academic environment does suggest that this is where retention programs will be most successful (Cope, 1987). Tinto (1987a) also found the most important variables were academic and social integration.

RETENTION OF NURSING STUDENTS

Pantages and Creedon (1978) asserted a correlation between persistence and fit between a student's attitudes and values and those of the institution. In order for students to create a fit in the system, congruence with the environment may mean the difference between persistence and withdrawal (Astin, 1984; Clarke, 1987; Pascarella, 1986; Tinto, 1975).

Persistence in college requires more than adequate adjustment; it also requires ". . . meeting of a number of minimum standards regarding academic performance" (Tinto, 1987b, p. 50). Tinto wrote that only 15 percent of all students depart from the institution as a result of academic dismissal. "Most departures are voluntary in the sense that they occur without any formal compulsion on the part of the institution" (Tinto, 1987b, p. 51). These voluntary departures, according to Tinto, result from incongruence between the student and the college environment; that is, a mismatch or lack of fit between the needs, interests, and preferences of the individual and those of the institution.

Positive institutional characteristics linked to retention were identified in a study by Beal and Noel (1980). They found that faculty-student interaction and a caring attitude of the faculty are among the most important reasons for student persistence. Academic advising was also linked to retention. Cowart (1987) found the caring attitude of faculty and staff, high quality of teaching, and academic advising to be among the top variables associated with student retention. Bajdek and Kim (1988) found that the single most important institutional factor that improves retention of college students is quality teaching.

Stodt (1987b) described the social environment as ". . . all non-academic programs and services, such as individuals who take a personal interest in students, financial support, adequate orientation programs, appropriate counseling services, and support systems that make students feel a part of the college community" (p. 21).

According to Tinto (1987), the social environment may include extra-curricular activities and day-to-day personal interactions among students, faculty, and staff which take place informally.

The Tinto (1987b) model includes the student's interaction with faculty outside the classroom, suggesting that such interaction not only increases social integration but also increases the individual's academic integration. A study conducted by Pascarella and Terenzini (1977) supported this concept. They concluded that ". . . informal student-faculty interaction is a significant predictor of college persistence" (p. 550).

Pascarella and Terenzini (1977) also found that the absence of interaction that enhances integration is likely to lead students to disassociate themselves from the college or university and eventually voluntarily withdraw. Noel (1987), supported this position and wrote, "Evidence mounts that experiences that promote the student's social and intellectual integration into the communities of the college are likely to strengthen their commitment and therefore reinforce persistence" (p. 25).

Tinto (1987b) asserted that persistence in college requires individuals to adjust not only intellectually but also socially to a new and somewhat strange world of college. Cope (1987) included faculty in the social system of the institution of higher education. He also maintained that social interaction with faculty is related to retention.

Implementation of retention strategies should be directed toward traditional student affairs programs and services (Webb, 1987) but should not be limited to that department. Retention of college students is the responsibility of the entire campus and is enhanced by a caring attitude of all members of the campus community.

METHODS

The purpose of this study was to determine if relationships exist between campus characteristics and retention of associate degree nursing students as perceived by their directors. It is hoped that this study may provide useful information about relationships between the nursing student and the college environment and, as a result, implicate changes that will enhance the retention of qualified students in associate degree nursing programs.

Retention of students in associate degree nursing programs is important not only to nursing educators but also to those in nursing service. Students enter these programs with intentions of being successful. The complex health care delivery system requires a larger number of more highly qualified nurses than ever before. Competent associate degree nurses are in great demand during this critical nursing shortage primarily because they are educated as bedside nurses. At a time when enrollment in nursing programs is lower than in previous years, providing an environment conducive to the successful completion of nursing education should be a priority for educators.

Research Questions

1. Is there a relationship between the retention/attrition rate in associate degree nursing programs and campus characteristics as rated by nursing program directors?
2. Is there a relationship between the description of systematic retention studies by associate degree nursing programs and campus characteristics as rated by nursing program directors?
3. Is there a relationship between the type of institution and campus characteristics as perceived by the directors of associate degree nursing programs?
4. What are the responses of the directors regarding action plans listed in the survey instrument as described by descriptive statistics?

The Instrument

This study utilized an adaptation of the instrument "What Works in Student Retention," a survey tool developed by Beal and Noel (1980), later revised by Cowart (1987), and further revised for this study. It was beyond the scope of this research to include this entire questionnaire. Questions related to dropout proneness and sections that address campus organization for retention and evaluation were excluded. Also, this study did not request the respondents to include samples of action plans. The type and control of the institution were added at the end of the questionnaire.

This project was designed to measure relationships between campus characteristics as perceived by nursing program directors and attrition rate, level of institutional involvement in retention, and type of institution. The instrument was mailed to a random sample of 250 National League for Nursing accredited associate degree nursing programs in the United States. A total of 185 nursing directors (74 percent) responded; however, only 180 (72 percent) of the questionnaires were usable.

The responses on the questionnaires were analyzed to determine not only frequencies but also to test for significant relationships through chi-square analysis. Since a large number of statistical tests were performed, a Bonferroni adjustment was performed for each hypothesis to confirm the results.

No other studies were found in the literature that specifically used this questionnaire. However, since it addresses positive as well as negative campus characteristics and was developed for distribution to administrators, it was chosen for this study.

Since no quantitative studies were found that used this instrument, reliability information is not available. In order to establish a measure of reliability, a Cronbach's Alpha, based on internal consistency, was performed.

RESULTS

Table 1 is a summary of the attrition rate of the programs as reported by the directors. An open-ended question was used on the survey instrument to gather this information. The reported rates were then ranked and divided into approximately three equal groups which were labeled Category I (low attrition), Category II (moderate attrition) and Category III (high attrition). Category I included 54 (31.77 percent), Category II had 60 (35.29 percent) of the programs, while the remaining 56 programs (32.94 percent) were placed in Category III. Ten of the directors did not respond to the question. The reported rates ranged from 0 percent attrition in some nursing programs to as high as 80 percent in others. The mean attrition rate was calculated to be 20.5 percent with a standard deviation of 14.92. Of the directors who responded to this question, 54.9 percent indicated this represented actual data while 45.1 percent stated the responses were based on estimated attrition rates.

In response to the questions relating to negative campus characteristics, the directors rated conflict between class schedule and job as the most important reason for students dropping out of their

Table 1
Attrition Rate as Reported by Directors of
Associate Degree Nursing Programs

Category	Total		Actual		Estimated	
	n	%	*n*	%	*n*	%
I: 0–10% attrition	54	31.77	32	34.4	22	28.9
II: 11–23% attrition	60	35.25	31	33.3	29	38.2
III: 24–80% attrition	56	32.94	30	32.3	26	32.9

N = 170; Range = 0% to 80%; M = 20.5%; SD = 14.92.

nursing programs (Table 2). The mean value was 3.69 on a scale of one to five. Fifty-six (31.6 percent) of the 180 directors rated this of highest importance and 57 (32.2 percent) rated this conflict of moderately high importance, while only 16 (9 percent) rated the conflict between class schedule and job of low importance. The second most important reason given for attrition was inadequate financial aid with 41 (23.3 percent) of the directors rating this of highest importance. The third most important reason, inadequate counseling support system, only had a mean value of 2.36, a rating actually of lower importance. Of the responses, 60 (34.3 percent) indicated lowest importance while 13 (7.4 percent) were highest importance. The directors indicated inadequate extra-curricular offerings to be the least important reason why students leave their programs. One hundred and twenty-five (71.4 percent) responded that this reason was of lowest importance. Restrictive rules and regulations governing student behavior was also believed to be of little importance as a reason for students not returning to their second year of the associate degree nursing program with 113 (66.3 percent) directors indicating it of lowest importance and only 2 (1.1 percent) rating it as highest importance. The third least important negative campus characteristic was unsatisfactory living accommodations with 71.1 percent (113) of the sample rating it as low importance.

Table 3 displays the responses to the questions that relate to positive campus characteristics and retention. The directors overwhelmingly believed that a caring attitude of faculty and staff was very important to retaining students from the first to the second year of the associate degree nursing program. Of the 180 responses, 133 (74.7 percent) indicated high importance. The mean score for this variable was 4.68 on a scale from one to five. Consistent high

Table 2
Negative Campus Characteristics and Attrition

Items (Item Numbers)	*M*
Conflict between class schedule and job (D.17)	3.69
Inadequate financial aid (D.7)	3.24
Inadequate counseling support system (D.5)	2.36
Inadequate academic support services learning centers, and similar resources (D.6)	2.31
Inadequate academic advising (D.4)	2.18
Inadequate part-time employment opportunities (D.8)	2.09
Inadequate career planning services (D.9)	1.83
Inadequate personal contact between students and faculty (D.14)	1.77
Inadequate opportunity for cultural and social growth (D.15)	1.75
Lack of faculty care and concern for students (D.1)	1.70
Quality of teaching not consistently high (D.3)	1.66
Lack of staff care and concern for students (D.2)	1.63
Insufficient intellectual stimulation or challenge (D.16)	1.61
Inadequate curricular offerings (D.11)	1.57
Unsatisfactory living accommodations (D.13)	1.57
Restrictive rules/regulations governing student behavior (D.12)	1.50
Inadequate extra-curricular offerings (D.10)	1.43

$N = 180$

quality teaching was also believed to be very important in retaining students with 96 (54.2 percent) rating this variable as very high importance. The third most important reason given by these directors was consistent high quality of academic advising. Fifty-eight (33 percent) rated this variable as high importance. Only 3 (1.7 percent) of the directors rated any of these top three campus characteristics as low importance as related to retaining nursing students. Encouragement of student involvement in campus life was not believed to be important to retaining student with only 11 (6.4 percent) giving it a high importance rating. Career planning services were not seen as an important retaining variable; 19 (10.8 percent) rated it important. Overall concern for student-institutional fit was not seen as an important positive campus characteristic related directly to retention of nursing students. Fifty-one (29.1 percent)

Table 3
Positive Campus Characteristics and Retention

Items (Item Numbers)	*M*
Caring attitude of faculty/staff (F.1)	4.68
Consistent high quality of teaching (F.2)	4.48
Consistent high quality of academic advising (F.3)	3.94
Adequate financial aid programs (F.4)	3.51
Admissions practices geared to recruiting students likely to persist to graduation (F.5)	3.51
Excellent counseling services (F.7)	3.50
System of identifying potential dropouts (F.9)	3.39
Overall concern for student-institutional "fit" (F.6)	3.21
Excellent career planning services (F.8)	3.11
Encourage student involvement in campus life (F.10)	2.50

$N = 180$

rated it as moderately high and 23 (13.1 percent) gave institutional fit a high importance rating.

The chi-square test statistic was used to test the null hypotheses. The results were organized in groups rather than looking at individual items. Negative and positive campus characteristics were grouped in order to enhance discussion of the data.

The six hypotheses tested in sub-problem 1 looked at the relationship between attrition rate and campus characteristics. Although none of the hypotheses were rejected, several significant relationships were found between attrition rate and the directors' perceptions and individual campus characteristics. Directors at programs with lower attrition rates do not place as much importance on the role of inadequate academic support services, learning centers, and similar resources as related to students leaving nursing programs. It was also found that more directors from programs with low attrition placed low importance on conflict between class schedule and job than programs with higher attrition rates. More directors from programs with high attrition believed that the conflict between class schedule and job was an important factor related to students dropping out of the nursing programs.

Sub-problem 2 dealt with the level of involvement in analytical study of attrition/retention and the directors' perceptions of the importance of campus characteristics. Several significant relationships were found when testing these six hypotheses. Directors of associate degree nursing programs who were involved in attrition/retention study gave higher ratings to several negative campus characteristics. They rated inadequate financial aid, conflict between class schedule and job, and insufficient intellectual stimulation or challenge higher than the directors who were not involved in retention. Those who were involved in study rated inadequate opportunity for cultural and social growth lower than the other directors. Directors who were not studying attrition/retention, but saw the need, rated inadequate support systems, lower importance. Inadequate academic advising and inadequate personal contact between faculty and students were rated lower importance by directors who were not studying attrition/retention and those who did not see the need for such analytical studies.

The only significant finding in sub-problem 3 was the relationship between the type of institution and the directors' rating of the importance of high quality academic advising as a positive campus characteristic related to retention of associate degree nursing students. More directors from colleges and universities rated this variable higher importance than the directors from community colleges and technical colleges.

Sub-problem 4 included a list of action plans in which the directors were asked to indicate if the plans had been implemented on their campuses. An overwhelming number of campuses have implemented programs that enhance the retention rate of the students.

DISCUSSION

Directors of associate degree nursing programs in the United States are concerned about retaining students from the first year to the second year of their programs. They indicated that conflict between class schedule and job was the most important reason for students leaving their programs. This finding is contrary to the administrators responses in both the Beal and Noel (1980) and the Cowart (1987) studies. Cowart (1987) found the most important reason was inadequate academic advising with conflict between class schedule and job ranking second. Beal and Noel (1980) found the most important factor in attrition was inadequate academic advising with conflict between class schedule and job ranking third.

More consistent results were found among the positive campus characteristics. This study of responses of nursing directors, the Beal and Noel (1980) study, and the Cowart (1987) study found caring attitude of faculty and staff and consistently high quality of teaching were the most important factors associated with retaining students in colleges and universities.

According to statistical analysis, an insufficient number of significant results were found in all of the 18 hypotheses tested. None of the hypotheses were rejected; however, significant findings were identified with chi-square tests on individual items. There does seem to be some relationship between attrition rate and the directors' perception of the importance of negative campus characteristics. The level of involvement seemed to be even more significant. Additional significant relationships were identified between involvement and the negative campus characteristics. Directors who were involved in attrition/retention studies rated conflict between class schedule and job and inadequate financial aid higher than the other directors. The directors who were involved in retention placed less importance on support systems and insufficient cultural and social growth. Also, the directors who were involved in study placed higher importance on having a system for identifying potential dropouts and those who were not studying attrition/retention rated financial aid higher than those who were involved in retention studies.

The majority of associate degree nursing programs in the United States are on campuses that have programs especially designed to enhance retention of students. This, coupled with the directors' interest and involvement in retention, may account for the lower attrition rates (mean=20.5 percent) in associate degree nursing programs as opposed to the overall attrition rate on two-year campuses (mean=47.8 percent) as documented by ACT (National Dropout Rates, 1991).

Associate degree nursing programs should clearly publicize the anticipated schedule of nursing classes prior to admission to the program. Alternative scheduling may be limited by the nature of the required clinical experiences and available clinical facilities as well as budgetary constraints. Additional research should be done in regard to the conflict between class schedule and job in view of the fact that there may be differences between nursing students and other students here. An attempt should be made to determine this difference in order to recommend possible remedies.

There seems to be a difference in the need for financial aid among nursing students. The directors, in their written comments, indicated the need for students to have additional funds to assist in meeting living expenses. Nursing directors should be aware of this difference and should be searching for additional assistance for the students. The development of on campus, low-cost child care would also benefit nursing students.

Since faculty concern for students is consistently seen as an important factor in the retention of students, nursing directors should nurture these relationships and provide opportunities for interaction between faculty and students outside the classroom. Academic advising was also seen as important and should be encouraged among the nursing faculty.

Nursing directors should reward quality teaching since this factor also has been consistently associated with retention of students. Quality programs are also more attractive to students according to written comments by the directors.

Additional quantitative research using this instrument would also be beneficial. Several significant relationships were identified in this study; however, the hypotheses were not rejected. Repetition of this study with other types of nursing programs would be helpful in determining the extent of this problem and in generalizing to programs other than associate degree nursing programs.

Because of the limitations of this study, generalizations cannot be made about all levels of nursing education. Further research using this instrument would provide valuable information regarding nursing education in general. Comparisons of various types of nursing programs would also be helpful in planning programs to enhance retention of nursing students.

REFERENCES

Astin, A. W. (1984). Student involvement: A developmental theory for higher education. *Journal of College Student Personnel, 25*(4), 297–308.

Bajdek, A. J., & Kim, S. (1988, July). *What makes students happy: A regression analysis of a recent student opinion survey at Northeastern University.* Paper presented at the National Conference on Student Retention, Boston, MA.

Cooper, C., & Bradshaw, R. A. (1984). How green is your academic climate? Check it with MOSS: A monitor of student satisfaction. *College and University, 59*(3), 251–260.

Cope, R. G. (1987). Why students stay, why they leave. In L. Noel (Ed.). *Reducing the dropout rate.* (pp. 1–11). San Francisco: Jossey-Bass.

Cowart, S. C. (1987). *What works in student retention in state colleges and universities.* Iowa City, Iowa: The American College Testing Program.

Meissner, J. E. (1986). Are we eating our young? *Nursing 86, 16*(3), 51–53.

National dropout rates: Freshman to sophomore year by type of institution. (1991). Iowa City, Iowa: The American College Testing Program.

Noel, L. (1987). Increasing student retention: New challenges and potential. In L. Noel, R. Levitz, & D. Saluri (Eds.), *Increasing student retention.* (pp. 1–27). San Francisco: Jossey-Bass.

Pantages, T. J., & Creedon, C. F. (1978). Studies of college attrition: 1950–1975. *Review of Educational Research, 48*(1), 49–101.

Pascarella, E. T. (1986). A program for research and policy development on student persistence at the institutional level. *Journal of College Student Personnel, 27*(2), 100–107.

Pascarella, E. T., & Terenzini, P. T. (1977). Patterns of student-faculty informal interaction beyond the classroom and voluntary freshman attrition. *Journal of Higher Education, 48*(5), 540–552.

Rosenfeld, P. (1988). Measuring student retention: A national analysis. *Nursing & Health Care, 9*(4), 198–202.

Stodt, M. M. (1987b). Intentional student development and retention. In M. M. Stodt & W. M. Klepper, (Eds.), *Increasing retention: Academic and student affairs administrators in partnership.* (pp. 15–26). San Francisco: Jossey-Bass.

Tinto, V. (1975). Dropouts from higher education: A theoretical synthesis of recent research. *Review of Educational Research, 45,* 89–125.

Tinto, V. (1987a). Dropping out and other forms of withdrawal from college. In L. Noel, R. Levitz, & D. Saluri (Eds.). *Increasing student retention.* (pp. 28–43). San Francisco: Jossey-Bass.

Tinto, V. (1987b). *Leaving college: Rethinking the causes and cures of student attrition.* Chicago: The University of Chicago Press.

Webb, E. M. (1987). Retention and excellence through student involvement: A leadership role for student affairs. *NASPA Journal, 24*(4), 6–11.

PART IV

Faculty and the Community: New Settings to Teach Contemporary Nursing Care

13

Gateway to the Caregiver: Collaborating to Meet the Needs of Education, Practice, and Community

Jeanne M. Novotny
Patricia P. Seymour
Susan J. Stocker

*I*n this paper, we share our experience in how our attempts to meet a community need evolved into what we believe will become part of our associate degree nursing curriculum. Our experience deals with the application of distance learning technology to reach caregivers in the home; the involvement of nursing students with these caregivers; the interaction of the community at large; the curricular implications for AD students in home care; and our vision for the future.

The community-based "Gateway to the Caregiver" program began when faculty identified a need of caregivers in the home for information and support in tending to their loved ones. After meeting with local nurses who had expertise in various aspects of home care, geriatrics, and psychiatric nursing, a planning committee was formed. Since our local campus was part of a distance learning link throughout our county, we used this technology to reach our target audience. Early in the planning process, we discussed the roles of the nursing student in providing home care. The following objectives served as a framework for our program:

1. Provide adult caregivers in Ashtabula County with accessible information about the prevention, identification, and management of common health problems that occur in the home.

2. Establish mechanisms that foster communication between caregivers to improve the quality of patient care.

3. Strengthen collaborative efforts among and between nurses, other professionals, and the greater Ashtabula County community.

4. Use the existing interactive television system to provide a cost-effective adult education program.

5. Identify the roles and competencies of the AD student nurse in relation to home health care.

6. Describe necessary curricular changes in the associate degree program to incorporate home health care.

DISTANCE LEARNING

Interactive television is one form of distance learning in which the majority of the instruction occurs while the educator and at least some of the learners are separated from one another at remote sites. By using a system of fiber optics and integrating television sets, fax machines, overhead projectors, and other equipment, students and instructors at geographically separate sites can see, hear, and interact directly with all other participants. This technology is available in our county and is accessed through our nine high schools, located throughout the county, and the local branch of Kent State University, located in the northern center of the county.

Ashtabula County, geographically the largest county in Ohio, is located in the northeastern section, approximately 50 miles between Cleveland, Ohio, and Erie, Pennsylvania. Despite its close proximity to major metropolitan areas, its population of just under 100,000 remains rural. The northern third of the county has the majority of the population base, which is located in three small towns; the rest is unequally dispersed throughout its approximately 700 square miles. In planning our adult focused program, we viewed the interactive television system (ITV) as one way to access potential participants who would otherwise not travel the distance to attend such a program.

After exploring the ITV system, we believed that it offered other benefits that were not available in a traditional classroom program setting. First, the system was available to us at no charge; since the project was nonfunded, the ITV system was an important consideration to both planners and participants. We would be able to provide this program free of charge to any interested adult. Secondly, participants could access the program quickly within their own community. Since adult caregivers often provide total care for their loved ones, they are infrequently able to attend outside programs due to restrictions on time and energy. Last, the speakers and planners were excited to explore this new technology and viewed the effort as a professional challenge.

We had some concerns about the complexities of using ITV with adult learners. Was the ITV system an appropriate delivery system for our program? Would participants at remote sites feel isolated and not fully involved? Would they be uncomfortable with the technology? According to one article, students have shown that live interactive television is as effective as face-to-face instruction (Hegge, 1993). The adult learner particularly benefits from interaction between and among students. With distance learning, the instructor must be cognizant of the psychological separation between teacher and students and between students at different sites and include this distinction in planning. We organized an orientation program for all speakers, which included familiarizing them with the technology and how to make the system user friendly for the participants. In addition, we selected volunteers who would be available at each site for the duration of the program. Some of the requirements we highlighted for speakers and site representatives included:

1. Assurance that participants at each site were addressed as if they were in the same room with the speaker.
2. Flexibility in room arrangement to encourage interaction among participants.
3. Availability of accessories, including fax machines, overhead projector, and videos, to vary educational approach and preserve learner interest.
4. Time for interaction and response throughout the presentation.
5. Awareness of the importance of television presence including dress, posture, and speaking hints.

As we continued our planning with community leaders for the "Gateway to the Caregiver" program, we were confident that the ITV system would help us meet our goal: to provide education and support to improve the quality of life of the homebound patient and caregiver. No one is more aware of the trends in health care reform than the family members who often become domestic caregivers. Such persons are frequently isolated and lack the education and support necessary to carry out this demanding role.

COMMUNITY COLLABORATION

In anticipation of even more sweeping changes in the health care system, we did not want to undertake this project in isolation. Both the *NLN Vision for Nursing Education* and *Nursing's Agenda for Health Care Reform* emphasize the importance of community and collaboration. Our faculty viewed this project as a means of beginning to build linkages between education and community. We began this collaborative effort by meeting with nurses from home health care, long term care, and other community agencies. We explained our idea, discussed the perceived needs of caregivers, and identified topics for presentation. Individuals enthusiastically volunteered to help plan the series of educational offerings, to assist with publicity, and to recruit caregivers. Others expressed an interest in serving as ITV site representatives, while still others agreed to present the weekly topics. The first "Gateway to the Caregiver" series was held in the fall of 1993. It was designed as six weekly sessions, each session one hour long. Caregivers attended the sessions at the ITV site nearest their home. The topics presented during this series included "Taking Care of Yourself," "Bridging Communication Gaps," "Home Care Tips," "Issues Related to Death and Dying," and "Community Resources." The participant evaluations were favorable. Respondents did, however, note that they required more time for informal interaction among the participants and presenters as a means of support. A second series was presented in the spring of 1994 and the weekly sessions were expanded to one and a half hours to accommodate this need.

In keeping with the collaborative spirit, we were pleased to be able to use the expertise of local nurses to provide the weekly presentations. Nursing faculty and nurses from the community served as co-presenters for some of the sessions. We believe our associate degree program is unique in that several of the faculty members have experience in home health care. However, inexperienced faculty members saw this moment as an opportunity for development.

They realized that home care nursing is simply not "acute care nursing in another setting," and that, if they are going to be asked to take students into these settings in the near future, they must be prepared.

As our project developed it became clear that respite care was an integral component. We used our nursing students to meet this need. This raised the following questions: What type of preparation would be necessary to send students into a home? Is it appropriate? How would their role be differentiated from the baccalaureate prepared nurse? How would faculty teach one more responsibility in an already intense curriculum?

COMMUNITY-BASED EDUCATION

Nursing education must of course provide appropriately prepared nurses who are able to function in a community-based, community-focused health care system (NLN, 1993). This shift in emphasis for all nursing education programs at all levels is new and has major implications for nursing education. The associate degree nursing program was originally designed to prepare a nurse who worked in a hospital in a well-defined, circumscribed nursing role. The intent of the program was to prepare graduates for the responsibilities commonly associated with registered nurses (Waters & Limon, 1987). It was assumed that associate degree nurses would work with baccalaureate nurses, who would perform at a level beyond that of the nurse with an associate degree. This assumption was incorrect for several reasons: (1) the number of associate degree nursing programs and the number of graduates increased much more rapidly than anyone expected and, (2) no substantive differentiation of work roles between ADN and BSN graduates developed in hospitals where, historically, most nurses have worked.

Based on our history, we need to explore new directions in associate degree nursing if we are to set the stage and shape our curricular endeavors to serve a rapidly changing society and workplace. In no way do we see associate degree nursing education abandoning the hospital or nursing home setting; in no way do we see associate degree nurses moving into roles for which they are unprepared or which infringe on baccalaureate and higher degree roles. What we do need is to differentiate between the practice roles in the work setting. Associate degree graduates are being employed in community agencies across the nation even when they are not prepared for this role. This is the ideal opportunity for nursing practice and education to collaborate in differentiating the roles of nursing in the work world.

The idea of using nursing students in our caregiver program was innovative and viewed with apprehension. However, we were committed to the venture and forged ahead. We felt that by establishing partnerships with family caregivers, students interested in home care would be able to gain an appreciation of the skills and understanding that the family brings to the caregiving situation. An extensive review of the literature revealed only one article (Hunt, Slette, & McKee, 1993) that dealt with community health concepts in associate degree nursing education.

We believe that the Caregiver Project has been transformational for those students who elected to become involved. One student, with the help of faculty, developed a questionnaire which was distributed to other students and faculty in order to elicit their ideas about how home care should be integrated into the curriculum. This student is now doing a poster session at a nursing conference. In addition, students who helped at the distance learning sites were able to participate in research and to present their experiences to peers. The students became excited about a project which was not rigidly controlled by faculty. Faculty found themselves reforming their ideas about how education should take place and about extending their repertoire of teaching skills. Education enriches and helps the learner grow in maturity and, in this case, the faculty shared in this transformation.

CONCLUSIONS

The Caregiver Project has given us the opportunity to form new partnerships with community agencies, to reach isolated caregivers, and to find new ways of educating students. Application of the new interactive television technology has been explored. We want to emphasize that we do not have the answers, but it is imperative that the nursing profession ask the questions and introduce new ways of learning. We have found the experience of trying something new exhilarating. Our expectation for the future is that associate degree educators will have the courage to try innovative ideas.

REFERENCES

Gallienne, R. L., Moore, S. M., & Brennan, P. F. (1993). Alzheimer's caregivers: Psychosocial support via computer Networks. *Journal of Gerontological Nursing, 19*(12), 15–22.

Barger, S. E. (1994). Educating nursing students for community-based practice. *Dean's Notes, 15*(3), 1–3.

Beach, D. L. (1993). Gerontological caregiving: Analysis of family experience. *Journal of Gerontological Nursing, 19*(12), 35–41.

Brugler, C., & Nypaver, J. (in press). Caregivers: Challenges and opportunities. *Journal of the American Hospital Association.*

Harrington, C. (1991). Why we need a teaching home care program. *Nursing Outlook, 30*(1), 10–13.

Harvath, T. A., Archbold, P. G., Stewart, B. J., Gadow, S., Kirschling, J. M., Miller, L., Hagan, J., Brody, K., & Schook, J. (1994). Establishing partnerships with family caregivers: Local and cosmopolitan knowledge. *Journal of Gerontological Nursing, 20*(2), 29–35.

Hegge, M. (1993). Interactive television presentation style and teaching materials. *The Journal of Continuing Education in Nursing, 24*(1), 30–42.

Hunt, R., Slette, E., & McKee, M. (1993). Community health concepts in associate degree curriculum. In J. Simmons (Ed.). *Prospectives: Celebrating 40 years of associate degree nursing education* (pp. 101–109) (No. 23-2527). New York: National League for Nursing Press.

Knight, B. G., Lutzky, S. M., & Macofsky-Urban, F. (1993). A meta-analytic review of interventions for caregiver distress: Recommendations for future research. *The Gerontologist, 33*(2), 240–248.

Lindgren, C. L. (1993). The caregiver career. *Image, 25*(3), 214–219.

Moore, A. J. (1981, November). *ADN education: A historical perspective.* Paper presented at the meeting, "Associate Degree Nursing: Achievements & Challenges, 1951–1981," Minneapolis, MN.

National League for Nursing. (1993). *A vision for nursing education.* New York: National League for Nursing Press.

National League for Nursing. (1991). *Nursing's agenda for health care reform.* New York: National League for Nursing Press.

Parkinson, C., & Parkinson, S. (1990). A comparative study between interactive television and traditional lecture course offerings for nursing students. *Nursing & Health Care, 10*(9), 499–502.

Pepin, J. I. (1992). Family caring and caring in nursing. *Image, 24*(2), 127–131.

Strauss, P. J., Wolf, R., & Shilling, D. (1992). *What every caregiver ought to know.* Chicago: Commerce Clearing House.

Waters, V., & Limon, S. (1987). Competencies of the associate degree nurse: Valid definers of entry-level nursing practice. (No. 23-2172). New York: *National League for Nursing Press.*

Wykle, M. (1994). The physical and mental health of women caregivers of older adults. *Journal of Psychosocial Nursing, 32*(3), 41–42.

Zartarian, S. *Benefits Analysis: Distance Learning.* Applied Communication Concepts, Inc., Research Triangle Park, NC.

Zink, M. R. (1989). Curriculum analysis of home health content in associate degree and baccalaureate degree nursing education. *Public Health Nursing, 6*(1), 8–15.

14

The Healing Web:
Curriculum Changes to Support
Differentiated Practice Roles
in the Community

June Larson
Susan Johnson
P. K. Holmes
Cheryl Leuning
Lois Schuller

As we near the turn of the century, it is important for nurses to take a thoughtful look at where we have been and where we are going. Debates surrounding health care reform have propelled nursing's agenda to increasing degrees of visibility and regard. Be that as it may, nursing still struggles with troubling internal issues. Entry into practice has been a divisive concept for over 30 years. Nursing's relationship with the medical community remains an on-going struggle for power and control. Important questions are being raised: Is there only one way and one place to learn? What kind of a nurse will be needed and how many will be needed? With the health care delivery system changing about us, how do we as educators respond to prepare our graduates to practice nursing appropriately?

The Healing Web (Figure 1) was born with these issues in mind. It began one afternoon over conversation. If we could work together, what would we envision doing together? What could we do? When could we get started? This partnership was also facilitated by the mutual valuing process already existing between the nursing service

Figure 1.   The Healing Web

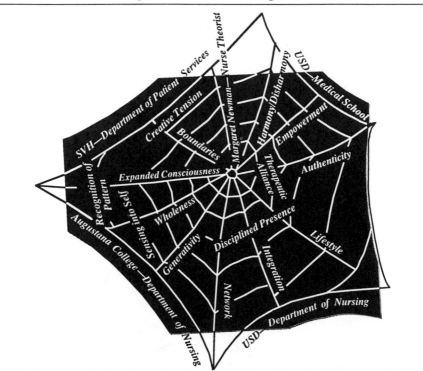

agency and the associate and baccalaureate nursing programs. Dialogue began over a shared clinical model for educating nurses to practice in the complementary roles of associate and primary nurses. Conversing together were a vice-president of patient services from the largest tertiary care center in the state, a chairperson and two faculty members from a private liberal arts college baccalaureate nursing program, and the chairperson and a faculty member from a public university associate degree nursing program.

The Healing Web is a consortium of these three organizations. This partnership is a collaborative effort designed to manage the transition from the present to the future of nursing education and practice. Students from the associate of arts nursing program at the University of South Dakota are working collaboratively with the baccalaureate nursing students from Augustana College to provide care to clients on a clinical unit within Sioux Valley Hospital's differentiated practice model. We have come together to form a partnership to facilitate educational preparation for the newly emerging and future nursing practice roles. Within this model, the associate student nurse provides comfort and physiological stabilization. The baccalaureate student nurse provides continuity of care and a timely discharge (Pitts-Wilhelm et al., 1991).

One of the most foundational concepts of the Healing Web is that of mutual valuing. Relationships which result in mutual valuing and respect can facilitate healing among health professionals. It requires that we value and embrace our diversity and the opportunities provided by our differences as well as our commonalities. The differences include our personal background, educational preparation, abilities, and domains of practice. Healing will result in a wholeness, and it is in coming to a full circle of wholeness that we can then embrace the differences. Trust is an essential component in building a true partnership where collaboration is the key to building an excellent model.

The core group of the Healing Web began meeting in 1990. In 1992, the partnership was formalized between the institutions by creating the Healing Web Institute. In 1993, the national healing web network was established, expanding the work of the Healing Web by bringing in others from Montana, Utah, Minnesota, Nebraska, California, and Wisconsin.

In Navaho culture, the legend of Spider Woman tells of her saving the people from a great flood by weaving a web on the surface of the water. People were saved by climbing onto the web and floating on it as if on a raft. Tradition also states that Spider Woman taught the Navajo people ways of helping them think clearly by creating the strings and designs of the web (Weigle, 1989). During changing times in health care such as we are now experiencing, it is important for nurses across the country to form alliances that allow us to understand each other, listen to one another and learn creative ways to work together. The Healing Web provides this kind of opportunity.

In the Healing Web Model, the role of the nurse is specifically defined and mutually valued. No one nurse or role is held in higher esteem than another. Integration, another core concept of the Healing Web, allows partners to relate in a mutual cooperative way. Relationships are collaborative rather than hierarchial. In the past, levels of nursing were represented as a hierarchial structure (Figure 2). At

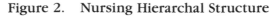

Figure 2.   Nursing Hierarchal Structure

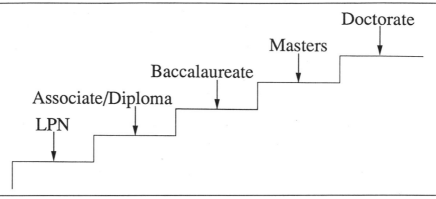

each level, the nurse was viewed as more powerful and better than those below. The Healing Web Model for the future is represented by a continuum (Figure 3). This model represents unity and inter-connectedness. The associate degree role is the common ground. As the nurse moves along the continuum, the complexity of function and emphasis in practice changes, yet the value and worth of each individual and each role is viewed as equal to others (Larson et al., 1992). Each is expert in the specified role and is part of the whole of nursing. With mutual valuing, collaboration, and integration, nurses begin to relate in a new and cooperative way that enhances

Figure 3.   The Whole of Nursing

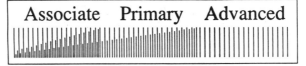

- **Each nurse is expert in the role**
- **Each role is mutually valued**
- **Collaborative practice utilizing all roles is the <u>whole</u> of Nursing Practice**

patient care and nurse satisfaction. Therefore the Healing Web project gives new vision to nursing education and service. It provides a framework to work together to weave a web of mutual valuing, trust and respect.

The Healing Web is a model for the reconciliation and transformation of nursing, designed to help education and service think more clearly about the future of nursing. Our relationships within nursing as well as medicine and other health care disciplines needs healing. We seek to begin the healing of wounds among nurses and between nursing and medicine. We have provided first-year students in the two nursing education programs and students in the first year of medical school the opportunity to meet for joint seminars to study issues of equal importance to all. We believe that in bringing the nursing and medical students together early in their education and providing them the opportunity to communicate and collaborate over a shared health care issue, we are beginning the process of healing. Collaborative relationships which result in mutual valuing, understanding, and respect can facilitate healing among nurses and between nurses and other health care professionals. Healing is defined as a process of bringing parts of oneself (physical, mental, emotional, spiritual, as well as relationships and choices) together at deeper levels of inner knowing, leading to an integration and balance, with each part having equal importance and value (Dossey, 1988).

A quote attributed to Chief Seattle, a great Native American leader, is an introduction to the Healing Web as metaphor and model:

> Woman did not weave the web of life, she is but a strand in it,
> Whatever she does to the web, she does to herself.

To the Healing Web core group, the web, with its characteristics of strength, healing, creativity, and clarity, seemed to fit as a model for the reconciliation and transformation of nursing education and practice and, ultimately, of health care. The model was created in the manner of the spider's weaving. The foundation lines include The University of South Dakota, Augustana College, and Sioux Valley Hospital. The bridge line from the center to the foundation lines was provided by Margaret Newman and her theory "Nursing as Expanding Consciousness." The radial lines are harmony, empowerment, authenticity, lifestyle, integration, network, generativity, wholeness, expanded consciousness, and boundaries (Bunkers et al., 1992). These concepts provide the foundation for the name Healing Web:

Harmony

Empowerment

Authenticity

Lifestyle

Integration

Network

Generativity

Wholeness

Expanded Consciousness

Boundaries

Caring is the primary focus of nursing efforts and includes a moral commitment to maintain the dignity of the client. The circular spiral lines in Figure 1 represent the expected outcomes or caring capacities of students educated in this model. These include sensing into self, disciplined presence, pattern recognition, therapeutic alliance, and creative tension. (Bunkers et al., 1992).

Pat Moccia has challenged us to "teach and learn with our students in those places where people live: in homes, communities, on the streets and in shelters" (Moccia, 1990). As we work to implement curriculum revisions to prepare the graduate to practice nursing in a health care environment we can only imagine, we are aware of the need to enable the graduate to make judgments and critical decisions in a variety of settings and nursing activities. The Healing Web is now beginning to move into the community with differentiated practice roles for the associate and baccalaureate nursing student. Our practice partners have expanded as we have begun to work with the Visiting Nurse's Association (VNA) in Sioux Falls. Typically when we tell the story of the Healing Web, we attempt to have at least two of our practice partners represented. As we began to plan for expansion of the project to include community, we paid conscious attention to building a partnership with the community agency.

PURPOSE OF COMMUNITY PROJECT

The purposes of the Healing Web Community Project are to provide the student the opportunity to: (1) develop skills in collaboration, critical thinking, and shared decision making; (2) view health and social issues as interactive; and (3) practice nursing in a community-focused health care system.

Objectives of Community Project

The associate nursing student will collaborate with a primary student to:

1. Assess the health status of the family.
2. Recognize how environment, culture, and socioeconomic status impact health and health care needs of families.
3. Identify the components of a therapeutic alliance.
4. Provide nursing care to individuals and families in the community setting following standards of practice for community health practice.
5. Identify family needs and communicate to primary nurse and instructor.

Differentiated Competencies in the Community

The following competencies were identified by the VNA, our community agency partner. They are adapted from the differentiated practice model in place at Sioux Valley Hospital (Koerner, 1989).

The collaborative community experience allows the nursing students the opportunity to know clients over time which provides them the much needed experience of continuity and consistency in the caregiver role. The students experienced first hand the lived experiences and needs of the clients in the community. Collaboration between the student practice partners provided the opportunity for collaborative decision making around a specific client care situation. We believe that those students educated in this model will be more skilled in continuity of care across the continuum. It is our belief that the learners will have a much clearer understanding and

Provision of Care (Technical Skills)

The student in the associate role manages care of clients.	The student in the primary role manages and integrates care for the client from admission to discharge.
Assesses and prioritizes the delivery of direct nursing care using time and resources effectively and efficiently.	Assesses and utilizes the nursing process to facilitate the delivery of holistic care using time and resources efficiently.
Performs nursing tasks/skills both legally and safely.	Performs/delegates skills both legally and safety.
Monitors/evaluates immediate patient responses to nursing and medical treatments.	Monitors, evaluates, and trends client responses to nursing, interdisciplinary team, problem list, medical treatments.
Delegates or refers aspects of care to health care team members consistent with their role and responsibilities.	Initiates and facilitates referrals to community resources.
Assumes responsibility and accountability for the direct nursing care and documentation.	Assumes responsibility and accountability for the direct care, caregiver effectiveness, and client outcomes.

Source: Adapted from the work of the Visiting Nurses Association, Sioux Falls, SD.

Communication (Interpersonal Skills)

The student in the associate role utilizes interactive communication.	The student in the primary role utilizes interactive communication.
Assesses the client to determine physical and emotional needs, as well as learning readiness.	Assesses the client's emotional needs and learning readiness with client's environment to develop a holistic plan of care.
Implements goal-directed interactions to encourage expression of client needs, supports safe client coping behaviors.	Facilitates goal directed interactions to promote effective coping mechanisms and necessary lifestyle changes.
Modifies, implements, and evaluates a teaching plan in order to restore, maintain, or promote health.	Designs, implements, and evaluates a holistic teaching plan that will maximize the client's potential for quality of life.

Continued

The student in the associate role utilizes interactive communication.	The student in the primary role utilizes interactive communication.
Cooperates with other members of the health team by communicating data based on nursing diagnosis to provide continuity of care.	Collaborates with other community resources to provide continuity of care.
Participates with other health team members in multi-disciplinary plans and problem resolution.	Assumes the role of change agent, consults and collaborates with other community resources to identify and resolve issues within the health care delivery system.

Source: Adapted from the work of the Visiting Nurses Association, Sioux Falls, SD.

Critical Thinking (Management Skills)

The student in the associate role manages care of clients.	The student in the primary role manages and integrates care for the client from admission to post-discharge.
Collects data from available resources utilizing established assessment format to identify basic care needs.	Expands the collection of data, using a holistic focus to identify health care needs.
Organizes and analyzes data to develop pertinent nursing diagnosis and related nursing care plan.	Analyzes and integrates complex data to develop further nursing problems.
Communicates with and involves the client to establish short-term goals that are consistent with the overall plan of care.	Uses foresight to negotiate long term goals with the client to develop a holistic plan of care.
Implements an individualized client plan of care using nursing diagnosis, policies, and procedures.	Implements and/or delegates a holistic plan of care utilizing a partnership commitment.
Evaluates client responses and modifies nursing interventions as necessary to meet client needs.	Evaluates progress toward established goals and promotes goal directed change to meet client needs.
Applies interpreted nursing research findings for nursing care.	Incorporates the research process to enhance nursing practice.

Source: Adapted from the work of the Visiting Nurses Association, Sioux Falls, SD.

acceptance of their own nursing roles as well as of those nurses whose educational preparation and expected role behaviors are different than their own. Learning experiences which are inherent in the Healing Web model lead to mutual valuing, collaboration and collegiality. It is our desire that the Healing Web is a healing experience for all who are involved in it.

REFERENCES

Bunkers, S., et al. (1992). The Healing Web: A transformative model for nursing. *Nursing & Health Care, 13*(2), 68–73.

Dossey, B. (1988). Nurse as healer: Toward the inner journey. In Dossey, B., Keegan, L., Guzzetta, D., & Kolkmeier, L., *Holistic nursing: A handbook for practice,* 39–53. Rockville: Aspen Publishers.

Koerner, J., et al. (1989). Implementing differentiated practice: The Sioux Valley Hospital experience. *Journal of Nursing Administration, 19*(2), 13–22.

Larson, J., et al. (1992). The healing web. A transformative model for nursing. *Nursing & Health Care, 13*(5), 245–251.

Moccia, P. (1990). No sire, it's a revolution. *Journal of Nursing Education, 29*(7), 307–311.

Pitts-Wilhelm, P., Nicolai, C., & Koerner, J. (1991). Differentiating nursing practice to improve service outcomes. *Nursing Management, 22*(12), 22–25.

Weigle, M. (1989). *Creation and procreation.* Philadelphia: University of Pennsylvania Press.

15

Community-Based
Maternal Child Nursing

Joanne Wit
Anne Miller

*I*n January 1993, it became apparent that the health care delivery system in Central Florida was beginning to evidence changes that reflected health care reform in our country. The Valencia Community College (VCC) nursing faculty had been looking at various curriculum changes that would include the community as client. We began to review the literature and look to our national organizations for trends and directions in nursing. The National League of Nursing (NLN) predicted and advocated that nursing education must include community learning experiences to meet the future health care needs of our country.

The NLN's October 1992 draft document, *Agenda for Nursing Education Reform,* calls for: "A shift in emphasis for all nursing education programs to ensure that all nurses—whatever their basic and graduate education and wherever they choose to practice—are prepared to function in a community-based, community-focused health care system. . . . An increase in the numbers of community nursing centers and their increased utilization as model clinical sites for nursing students. . . . An increase in the number of nursing faculty prepared to teach for a community-based, community-focused health care system."

The VCC nursing faculty undertook a project to include community into the curriculum. In addition to the NLN draft report, the faculty relied on the Pew Health Professions Commission report issued in 1993—*Health Professions Education for the Future and Schools in*

Service to the Nation. Their report stated, "The commission notes that a clear trend is emerging toward having nurses take on increasingly specialized tasks in primary care, highly specialized care and administration."

Another quote from this report states that, "As the pressures for more cost- and consumer-responsive health care mount, they will be, in part, translated into greater demand for community-oriented care. This will require health care professionals who are able to work with the broad array of social service providers in the community and are able to link together teams that can effectively focus on patient care needs."

The commission, while acknowledging the involvement of the nursing profession in Public Health nursing for over forty years, finds that, "This area of strength in nursing has not become the predominant theme in nursing practice or the delivery of nursing care. This resource will be invaluable to the nation's health care system as it struggles to address community needs."

THE NEW ENVIRONMENT

There was little research on the use of community setting versus the acute setting for educating associate degree nurses. Some information was available on adapting nursing curriculum to include outpatient community-based experience. We were on our own to test this new environment.

Currently, there are 1,400 schools of nursing in the United States.

Diploma	12 percent all programs
Associate Degree	50 percent all programs
Baccalaureate	38 percent all programs

Associate Degree programs enroll over one half of all students preparing to become RNs. A majority of the nursing work force is provided by associate degree nurses. The importance of this data is the fact that the nurses needed for community health practice will have to come from this large pool.

Most of nursing education lags behind current community-based practice. With new public policy and implementation of funding strategies expected to be in place, soon nursing education will lag even further behind unless changes are made to prepare nurses to serve in the increasing number of community-based practice settings. To meet this need, Valencia nursing faculty believe that nursing educators must broaden and refocus their knowledge base and educate future associate degree nurses in a responsive way. This project was a beginning to building a new knowledge base, changing the nursing curriculum, and identifying the settings in which teaching occurs.

In our community, Valencia graduates are hired in the acute care setting, but the number of entry positions has declined in the last few years. At the same time, positions in community-based settings are increasing in number and agencies are having difficulty filling their vacancies.

In order to get a realistic view of our community's needs and their input into the education of nurses, a day-long planning meeting was held with community-based providers in Orlando, in March of 1993, to determine the educational needs of nurses hired by these providers.

The providers who attended this planning session shared a troubling picture, revealing that to function well in the community-based setting all nurses need additional preparation in community nursing. Curriculum must include both content and strategies that will produce a nurse that has the specific qualities to do community nursing. The members of the planning committee generated the following list of desirable outcomes for associate degree graduates.

A program should be designed to:

1. Encourage critical thinking.
2. Enable graduates to collaborate with others in health care and social work teams.
3. Teach shared decision making.
4. Enable graduates to function in less controlled environments than the hospital.
5. Promote autonomy.
6. Strengthen graduates' assessment skills.
7. Involve graduates with health care needs of different communities.
8. Prepare graduates for prevention and wellness.

9. Prepare graduates for the differences in financing of community-based care.

The community-based providers also described a gap between what is taught in nursing schools and the reality of work situations in the community. The planning group members called for nursing educators to incorporate models of work settings in institutions that reinforce the use of skills needed in the community-based workplace upon graduation.

THE MATERNAL CHILD NURSING PILOT PROJECT

With preliminary work completed, a decision was made to use Maternal Child Nursing as our pilot in the community project. This practice specialty in nursing was chosen for a number of reasons. The following list depicts some of the faculty's thinking:

1. Increasingly instructors are finding it difficult to find pediatric and maternal newborn clinical placements.
2. Children are discharged sooner and sicker from the hospital.
3. Mother/newborn experience is limited because of 23 hour and even 6 to 12 hour discharges after delivery.
4. Students have problems related to experiencing continuity of care.
5. In many teaching hospitals, children are frequently too acutely ill to be cared for by nursing students.
6. Pediatric patients experience short-term hospitalization which leads to little time to assess growth and development.
7. Student assignments may not be appropriate where family is coping with an acute illness.
8. There is little time or exposure to learn about and teach health promotion behaviors.

We found that the community offered us a unique setting and environment in which to teach students. We also discovered that the clinical laboratories in our community were flexible, and the staff was very interested in taking on this responsibility. There were also many settings and experiences that could not be found in hospital-based clinical education.

Skilled in family systems, the Maternal Child Health faculty was chosen to begin the pilot. In the design of this project, agencies that provide community-based care were contacted to determine their willingness to accept the ADN student within their practice and a community role in the ADN educational process. The response was overwhelmingly positive. Some of our community health providers are beginning to offer employment and orientation programs to both ADN and BSN graduates. Their earlier policies of not hiring nurses who had not had at least a year of experience in acute settings is changing. We believe that if we produce nurses better prepared to work in this environment, hiring policies will change to an even greater extent.

The other major piece of this project was our work for approval with the state Board of Nursing. We presented the project to the board and received approval for a pilot. There was some debate over using the agency's nurse in the community as a preceptor before the completion of all didactic and clinical experience in the program of study. It was decided that the preceptor would be called a clinical associate with certain criteria required.

The pilot project was offered first in the summer of 1993 with two of the eight clinical groups in the Maternal Child Nursing course registered randomly into the experimental clinical experience. Two of the remaining six clinical groups served as controls.

The project was developed to answer four questions.

1. Will the student in Maternal Child Nursing meet the course theory and clinical objectives when the clinical experience includes a community-based experience?
2. Will a community-based experience increase the students' knowledge of community health agencies?
3. Will a community-based experience increase the value students place on the role of community health agencies?
4. Will the maternal child nursing student transfer learned skills to the community setting?

With these questions in mind and with state approval secured, the initial work to secure the clinical placements for the students was started. Selection of clinical facilities was based on several factors.

First, the experience had to promote the students' achieving the course objectives that were consistent with the philosophy and conceptual framework of the Nursing Program. Second, the clinical experience had to provide information that would answer the research questions. A packet was developed to present to the clinical sites that had been selected for use in the project. The packet consisted of the proposal presented to the state, the four research questions, clinical objectives for the students, skills already accomplished in previous nursing courses and those to be learned during the semester. The courses already completed were Fundamentals of Nursing and Basic Medical Surgical Nursing. With the packet in hand, we visited each of the clinical settings that had been selected. All of the facilities were being used by Valencia's nursing program in some capacity; therefore, we already had contracts and did not have to deal with this aspect of securing a clinical placement. We spoke with the nurse in charge of the unit, clinic or agency. As we explained the project, the clinical experience, and the objectives the students were to meet, we sought to convey the excitement we felt about this project and its impact on nursing education and our graduates. In response, the nurses gave enthusiastic support to our proposal. In some cases, we had to write or visit administrative personnel responsible for making the decision about our proposed clinical experience. In each case, full approval was given.

The sites chosen met the criteria that the student would be able to learn the nurse's role in health maintenance and wellness promotion and a registered nurse worked in the setting and was available to act as clinical associate. The sites chosen were a high-risk OB clinic; pediatric and prenatal clinics, both hospital-based and at the Public Health Department; an outpatient pediatric surgery clinic; a pediatric oncology clinic; a pediatric respite care, Family Practice Clinic; a Family Health Center providing care for an under-served population of migrant workers; and a private OB-GYN office. It is evident that the sites chosen offered structured settings with registered nurses to provide supervision to the associate degree nursing student and very different experiences.

Students' Clinical Experience

The day-to-day handling of the students' clinical experience was discussed individually with the nurse in each setting to set up a working relationship that would meet our objectives. The students were to be assigned to a setting for a three-week clinical experience. In most cases, this meant one 8-hour-day per week. The students were actively involved in the role of the nurse in that setting, within the limitation of skills already learned as part of the nursing program. This represented a change from previous use of these facilities. Before planning the pilot experience, the students spent four hours at many of these same facilities in an observational experience. Now the nurse in the setting would be responsible for student supervision and would participate with the instructor and students in evaluating clinical performance. The instructor would visit the clinical setting each week and be available by beeper if the nurse or the students needed to contact the instructor.

The clinical hours for the course were usually 10 hours per week. With an 8-hour clinical day, two hours each week were available for pre- and post-conferences which were held on campus. During the conference, the students shared their experiences. Even though the settings had a basic commonality, they were in fact very different. The students each did something different, but discovered that they were all accomplishing the clinical objectives. A common thread that permeated all experiences shared by the students included the teaching they found themselves doing and the opportunity they had to promote wellness.

As instructors, we found that our role was very different in the community setting. For the first three weeks of the clinical rotation the students were in the acute care setting. This time was planned very carefully to enable the students to meet the clinical objectives that could only be met in that setting and to prepare them to go into the community setting. When we left the hospital clinical, our role changed. We found ourselves functioning more as mentors. In our visits with the students, our role was to point out the learning they could do, how they could go about increasing their participation in the nurses' role in this setting, sharing with them that they did in fact have the basic building blocks to work in the setting. We also spent time with the nurse reinforcing the student role and the benefits to the students and the outpatient setting, and the patient as the student became knowledgeable in the community aspect of patient care. By the third week, the students were functioning as part of the staff with the clinical associate providing supervision. What did they do? They did some if not all of the following: intake interviews and assessments of antepartal clients, PPDs, immunizations, triage in pediatric clinic, taught classes in clinic waiting rooms, measured fundal height, assessed FHTs, tube feedings, trach suctioning, straight caths, assessed growth and development, learned why compliance is difficult for some clients, answered questions and provided teaching. We provided direct supervision in one area: administration of immunizations at the Public Health Department. The policy for all students at the Public Health Department facility was that they may only perform intrusive procedures with the supervision of an instructor. This meant one instructor for two students. We made the decision that it was worth it for one morning of the three-week experience. All other settings allowed the student to perform all skills with the supervision of the clinical associate. This was a step that we knew we would have to take from the very beginning and was incorporated as part of the experience when it was developed. To actually do it, however, was difficult. At first, in visiting each setting, I, for one, felt awkward, sometimes not needed, but with each visit and as the first week ran into the second week, I found that I had let go of what I had perceived as my role. I was moving to mentor and could feel comfortable with the supervision provided by the clinical associate and with the level of functioning of my students. I had to trust them as well as the faculty who taught the first two courses in the program. They had taught and evaluated many of the skills these students were now putting to use in the community setting. With my weekly visits to the students in the various settings, and in pre- and post-conference, I was able to see the students grow. They learned to trust their knowledge base, knew what they could and could not do, and began to know what autonomy meant. Critical thinking on the part of the students became evident as they discussed their experiences in pre- and post-conference.

At the end of the clinical experience, the clinical associate, student and I completed the clinical evaluation tool used for all students in the course. To receive a passing grade for a nursing course, a satisfactory clinical evaluation was necessary. This was also implemented for the students in the pilot clinical experience.

The intent of including the community experience in the Maternal Child Health Nursing course was to provide the student with the opportunity to observe and perform assessments and screenings, provide patient and family education and transfer skills previously learned and evaluated in the hospital and/or college laboratory setting. Student evaluations and pre-post test differences demonstrated a positive and enhanced learning experience. Students in the clinic settings performed as well as the other students. They showed an increased understanding and value of community-based settings and learned skills were transferred to the community setting.

An unexpected outcome of the project was that it allowed for increased interaction between the college's nursing faculty and nurses in community settings. This interaction helped bridge the gap that often exists between nursing education and nursing service. The community-based clinical associates expressed a great deal of satisfaction with their role in this project and encouraged the college faculty to continue the program after the pilot project ended.

We again offered the community-based clinical experience in the fall of 1993 and expanded it to four clinical groups during the summer of 1994. Valencia Community College is in the process of curriculum change in response to changes in health care delivery. The community is an arena we are exploring for educational experiences for our students. This pilot project provided valuable data in use of the community in the educational program of the Associate Degree nursing student.

The community experience is still offered. Each semester, we look at and use new facilities, including schools, pediatric emergency departments, birthing centers, and home care. As new settings come to our attention, we learn how to better facilitate the student's experience. A criterion that is always taken into consideration in placing students into a setting is that it prepares them for a role that is appropriate for the associate degree nurse. As we continue with our curriculum revision, we must keep our objective clear: To provide educational experiences that enable the student to assume an effective nursing role in the changing health care delivery system.

REFERENCES

American Nurses Association. (1990). *Nursing's agenda for health care reform, executive summary*. PR 12-91.

Haussler, S. C., & Cherry, B. S. (1993). The community: A primary site for students in pediatric nursing. *Journal of Nursing Education. 32.* (4), 183–184.

National League for Nursing. (1992). *An agenda for nursing education reform: In support of nursing's agenda for health care reform.* (draft)

Pew Health Professions Commission, (1993). *Health professions education for the future and schools in service to the nation.*

16

Senior Students and Senior Citizens: Reciprocal Benefits in Learning and Caring

Marcia F. Miller

*P*lacement of students in an extended care facility for clinical experience is not a new phenomenon. Usually the student is just beginning a program of study in nursing. The extended care setting is used by instructors to reinforce concepts that include body mechanics, nursing process, hygiene, nutrition, and aging. In the past 15 years, studies have been done that considered the use of these facilities for the clinical experience of senior students.

The addition of gerontological concepts and of nursing care centers in clinical practice has been examined by faculty across the country. For several reasons, the decision to schedule students into extended care facilities during their final weeks of study is difficult for many faculty to accept. Discussions center around any benefit to the students who may or may not choose to practice in such settings after graduation. Would students be able to practice and enhance the skills learned from previous classes? Would they be equipped to enter the field of nursing in a variety of clinical settings? There are no ready answers. The interests and capabilities of the students coupled with their educational preparation certainly influence their successes in employment. For the faculty making curricular decisions, one answer may be to offer a choice to those students who express an interest in caring for the older adult and the frail elderly.

Such is the case in the Associate Degree Nursing Program at Sinclair Community College in Dayton, Ohio, where students are being given the opportunity to choose between a hospital setting or an extended care facility in their final clinical rotation. For several years, students have completed their studies with a course designed to increase clinical practice prior to graduation. This course, Directed Nursing Practice, provides the opportunity to enhance technical skills under the guidance of an experienced registered nurse who acts as preceptor in the clinical setting. The majority of students spend eleven or twelve weeks assigned to a medical or surgical nursing unit in a local hospital working closely with the RN.

The quarter begins with the student shadowing the registered nurse as the student learns the role of the nurse in the hospital setting. The nurse is seen interacting with patients and family members, with peers and other health care providers. The nurse shares his or her knowledge and experience as the student is guided into the work setting. Next the student accepts responsibility for the care of two or three patients. Working on technical skills and on time management, the student gradually increases the patient numbers until the RN's daily assignment is carried by the student. At this point, the student is functioning as a primary caregiver with minimal guidance by the RN and instructor.

During the quarter, theory in the classroom is focused on concepts of time management, prioritization, decision-making and delegation. Nursing management and leadership within the hospital structure are examined. The student learns what to expect as he or she moves into the world of hospital nursing.

A variation of this course will take some senior students into an extended care facility for Directed Nursing Practice. Students are given the option of adding a clinical variation that incorporates the concepts of time management and prioritization with care of the older adult and the frail elderly and socialization into the profession of nursing in a nursing center or extended care facility.

Course content and clinical objectives are the same in both the hospital and the extended care facility. Learning experiences differ depending on the setting. Course objectives that are applicable to both settings include the expectation that the student will be able to:

- Practice nursing in either the acute care or the subacute care setting;
- Discuss the roles and responsibilities of the registered nurse in the hospital and in the extended care facility recognizing the differences and similarities in the roles;

- Use the nursing process in identification of patient/resident needs and in appropriate intervention;
- Manage the care of a group of patients or residents implementing principles of time management, prioritization, and decision making;
- Evaluate the effectiveness of communication techniques in both the hospital and the extended care facility;
- Demonstrate accountability by applying previously learned knowledge to the care of patients/residents.

The student spends six or seven weeks in the hospital setting working with an RN preceptor. Here the focus is on development of the skills of time management, priority setting, decision making, and delegation under the watchful eye of the experienced registered nurse.

In the final four or five weeks, students are sent to an extended care facility where they become members of a team providing care for a group of residents. Here the RN is role model and preceptor as the students rotate through positions of team leader and resident care manager. Students assess and revise the time management skills practiced in the hospital. Also, they have the opportunity to apply principles of decision making and delegation with peers and with nursing assistants.

Residents and members of the nursing home staff are eager partners in this program. A well-planned orientation for the nurses, nursing assistants, and support personnel in the nursing center is very important in setting the stage for a successful learning experience. The registered nurses are anxious to assist the students in learning about the similarities and differences in the work that they do and that done by their colleagues in the hospital. While nursing assistants are reluctant to accept the students into the hierarchy of caregivers at first, they do respond as they get to know the students and to understand the role of education in the facility. Residents are accepting of the students and are appreciative of the interest, attention, and care shown by them.

In this program, the current focus is on the role of the nurse in both the acute and the subacute care settings. The care of the older adult and the frail elderly individual is examined within the student's assignment. Concepts of gerontological nursing are not emphasized in the course content. Since many hospitalized patients are over seventy years of age, the students are able to apply variations in care needed by this age group and to examine those gerontological concepts through use of daily journal entries, interactions with instructor and registered nurse and through post conference processing of a day's events.

As the quarter ends, students express confidence in their ability to begin to work in either an acute care setting or in an extended care facility (ECF). While some say they will not seek employment in an ECF, all come away from the experience with a greater understanding of the needs of the older adult and an appreciation for the nurses who choose to work in extended care.

REFERENCES

Burke, M., & Sherman, S. (Eds.). (1993). *Gerontological nursing: Issues and opportunities for the twenty-first century.* New York: National League for Nursing Press.

Culley, J., & Courtney, J. (1993). Gerontology as a focus for traditional and nontraditional approaches to nursing education. In C. Herne (Ed.), *Determining the future of gerontological nursing education,* (pp. 87–88). New York: National League for Nursing Press.

Mezey, Lynaugh, & Cartier. (1988, November/December). The teaching nursing home program, 1982–1987: A report card. *Nursing Outlook,* pp. 285–292.

Verderber, & Kick. (1992, October). Gerontological curriculum in schools of nursing. *Journal of Nursing Education,* pp. 355–361.

Waters, V. (Ed.). (1992). *Teaching gerontology.* New York: National League for Nursing Press.

17

Pediatric Clinical Experience: Preparation for the Twenty-First Century*

Linda Rieg
Phyllis Augspurger

*O*ne strength of nursing education has been its continued use of hands-on practice-based clinical experience for students. Clinical experience allows the student the opportunity to see the textbook come to life and to practice skills under supervision. In addition, clinical experience exposes the student to the many roles of the nurse and socializes him or her into the profession. As the focus of health care changes, preparing the nurse for the next century necessitates changes in the traditional clinical experience at all levels of education. The traditional concentration of clinical experiences within an acute care setting needs to be restructured to include the expanding future roles of the nurse and the changes in the health care structure. The need for restructuring led us to adopt an organizational design for our pediatric clinical experience that was not at all traditional.

Nursing's Agenda for Health Care Reform (1991) supports restructuring the health care system to be proactive rather than reactive. Preventive health care is a major concept, a concept long advocated by nursing. Although nursing education had given lip service to preventive care, we still rely on the acute care setting for

---

*Reprinted with permission from the *Journal of Nursing Education*.

most of our clinical experiences. Reilly and Oermann (1992) agree and argue that this has continued despite the increasing complexity of the hospitalized patient.

Most professionals also agree that the setting for health care in the 21st century will change from the hospital to the home and community. Nurses have traditionally been involved in both these areas and should take a leadership role in the new system. Just as with preventive concepts, we talk about home- and community-based nursing care to basic nursing students but provide them with relatively few opportunities to experience this type of nursing.

Nursing leaders have called for a curriculum revolution in nursing education. The National League for Nursing's *Vision for Nursing Education* (1993) proposes that "educational experiences will be increasingly planned where people are—in the home, schools, and work sites, and in the ambulatory settings, long term-care facilities, in shelters and community gathering places—as well as in hospitals" (p. 11).

Nursing faculty have the power to influence the future direction of nursing. Most of us can recall one or more faculty members whose ideals, philosophy, or interests have influenced the direction our nursing practice has taken. In a recent article on nursing education, de Tornyay (1993) states "nursing faculty can and do influence the health care system through controlling what they teach, being role models, and by the clinical sites we choose for student experiences" (p. 302). Others have urged nursing educators to realize that there are many paths to follow in nursing education to produce the variety of nurses needed for the future. For example, Allen (1990) argues that our conformity to a single vision for nursing education has not produced creative and critical thinking nurses.

If nurses need to function in the community away from the acute care hospital, nursing educators must prepare them for that role in their basic educational preparation and not just in one course entitled Community Nursing. Indeed, some educators have reported successful use of community resources during the initial pediatric experience. Haussler and Cherry (1993) urged the use of the community as a primary site for teaching pediatric nursing. Streubert (1989) used a high school setting as an opportunity for students to assess and interact with adolescents, an experience missing from their hospital exposure.

CLINICAL EXPERIENCE

In an associate degree (AD) nursing program, the appropriateness of nonacute care clinical experience for students has been questioned. Some would argue that the AD nurse should only be prepared for acute care hospital positions. Nonetheless, we think that because of the trends in nursing and health care, we would be remiss to expose our students only to hospital-based care. Consequently, we reviewed the pediatric clinical experience in our program with a creative and critical eye. Our dilemma was to maximize the learning potential of the clinical experience and prepare our graduates to function in the future. We wanted to make every minute in the clinical experience valuable and relevant to the student.

The emphasis in our pediatric course has always been on the illnesses unique to children, the normal growth and development, preventative care, family dynamics, and normal childhood problems. Meeting these objectives in an acute care setting had become increasingly difficult. In our program, the pediatric course is seven weeks long in the first semester of the second year. We have a practicum of 12 contact hours per week which we had previously divided into two six-hour days spent in a children's hospital. We restructured the clinical time to include one eight-hour day in the hospital focusing on acute illnesses and the remaining four hours were devoted to normal growth and development and community field experiences. This format allowed the student to devote one third of his/her clinical time to health promotion and normal childhood development—concepts that are more congruent with our course objectives.

The hospital day was traditionally structured. Students were assigned to give complete care to one patient. Each week the student completed a clinical worksheet that included an in depth assessment, explanation of pathophysiology, drug therapy, other treatments, and an evaluation of the child's growth and development. All this data resulted in a nursing care plan designed specifically for the assigned child and family. This day also socialized the student into the role, responsibilities, and routines of the acute care hospital nurse.

The seven additional days were comprised of five classroom days and two field experiences. A variety of teaching/learning techniques were used during the laboratory days. One of our objectives was to involve the student in the process and give him/her the opportunity to think through problems in a nonthreatening environment. Traditional teaching techniques were limited to brief lectures and videos on hospitalization of children and normal growth and development. Participatory techniques such as case studies, problem solving in small groups, games, and computer assisted instruction (CAI) were used. The case studies, problems solving, and CAI programs allowed the students to make clinical decisions in a safe environment. Games such as Infant Jeopardy and Preschool Pursuit facilitated team building while at the same time drew upon their knowledge of growth and development. Inclusion of CAI in actual class time helped enable the students to become comfortable using the computer since this class would be taking CAT-NCLEX.

Objectives for the two field experiences included introducing the student to different environments for nursing care, observing preventative measures in action, observing growth and development, and seeing the variety of roles nurses assume. One field experience was in the ambulatory care center of the children's hospital. Students were assigned to either a neurology, dermatology, ENT, or a primary care baby clinic. The student was provided the opportunity to observe normal growth and development, common childhood illnesses, and the role of the nurse in the clinic. The other field experience was either with a home health nurse or a school nurse. In the school, the student observed the types of care given and the role of the nurse in the school. The home health visit provided the student the opportunity to see the complex care given in the home, the importance of family teaching prior to discharge, and the family/nurse dynamics in the home setting.

EVALUATION

Although no clinical experience will be evaluated positively by all students, the evaluations of the revised clinical schedule and particularly of the field experiences were generally enthusiastic. Even though we stress the role of the nurse as a teacher in the acute care setting, it is sometimes overshadowed by the technical tasks. Students were amazed that nurses in these community-based environments spent so much time teaching families rather than keeping busy doing things to patients.

Students were overwhelmed by the amount of acute care that was actually done in the home. Although some preferred the relaxed atmosphere of home care, others expressed discomfort with the slower pace. The involvement of the family in the care of the child became apparent to many students; they commented about the family's ability to do all of the technical tasks. They also noted the long-term personal involvement of many of the nurses in the care of these children. One student stated the experience was "an eye opener about how one's life must totally change when one has a child with a chronic illness."

Students who observed at schools were impressed with the screening and teaching activities of the nurses. One student helping with vision screening actually discovered she needed glasses. Students were astonished to find so many chronically ill and disabled children in the general school population. One observed two spina bifida children who needed to catheterize themselves and another, a child who suctioned herself. Students commented about the number of children with attention deficit disorder, a condition we rarely see in the hospital. Finally, one student observed the nurse in a collaborative role leading a group discussion of professionals and parents about solutions for a lead poisoning problem.

Students in the clinic also had a variety of experiences. In the neurology clinic students reported observing complex neurological exams and evaluation of seizure medications. Dermatology clinic gave them the opportunity to see skin disorders we normally do not see in the hospital. Ear, nose, and throat clinic provided a chance to see PE tubes and otitis media. Finally, the primary care clinic gave the students a chance to see nurses teach normal growth and development and administer immunizations. The comments of the students convinced us that seeing or experiencing the real thing could replace hours of traditional classroom teaching. Students gained insight into other roles for nurses and the importance of the prevention and health promotion aspects of the nurses' responsibilities.

An unexpected reward of this organizational design was the involvement of part-time clinical faculty in classroom situations. In addition to the full-time faculty, we rely on clinically excellent part-time faculty to instruct students in the hospital. One of the problems with this arrangement was the lack of communication between the full-time and part-time faculty and thus a potentially disjointed curriculum. We found that including the part-time faculty in the planning and execution of the laboratory day gave them the opportunity to test the educational waters by addressing a larger group of students. At the same time, it gave the full-time faculty time to talk with the part-time faculty to discuss problems and issues that may have occurred in the clinical setting. It was also an excellent opportunity to mentor young faculty and encourage them to continue their interest in education.

CONCLUSION

Although we reduced the amount of actual time in the hospital, we concluded that the additional experiences and variety of settings have enhanced the quality of our course. Course evaluation confirmed our belief that this organizational change enhanced the students' learning experience by giving them the opportunity to observe normal growth and development, preventative health care measures, and the role of the nurse outside the acute care setting. As nursing's focus changes and nursing meets the challenges of the twenty-first century, the faculty must address these changes now to prepare our students for the future. Students must be ready, even at the associate degree level, to fill the many roles that nurses will hold in the future. As de Tornyay states and we agree, nursing faculty can and so influence the future of health care through their teaching, role modeling, and clinical site selection.

REFERENCES

American Association of Colleges of Nursing. (1993). *Nursing education's agenda for the 21st century: A position statement.* Washington, DC.

Allen, D. (1990). The curriculum revolution: Radical re-visioning of Nursing Education. *Journal of Nursing Education, 29*(7), 312–316.

de Tornyay, R. (1993). Nursing education: Staying on track. *Nursing & Health Care, 14*(6), 302–306.

Haussler, S., & Cherry, B. (1993). The community: A primary site for students in pediatric nursing. *Journal of Nursing Education, 32*(4), 183–184.

Infante, M., Forbes, E., Houldin, A., & Naylor, M. (1989). A clinical teaching project: Examination of a clinical teaching model. *Journal of Professional Nursing, 5*(3), 132–139.

National League for Nursing. (1993). *A vision for nursing education.* New York: National League for Nursing Press.

Reilly, D., & Oermann, M. (1992). *Clinical teaching in nursing education.* 2nd ed. New York: National League for Nursing Press.

Streubert, H. (1989). An alternate pediatric clinical placement. *Journal of Nursing Education, 28*(5), 230–231.

Other Books of Interest from NLN Press

You may order NLN books by • TELEPHONE 800-NOW-9NLN, ext. 138
• Fax 212-989-3710 • MAIL Simply use the order form below

Book Title	Pub. No.	Price	NLN Member Price
☐ **Health Professionals Stylebook: Putting Your Language to Work** *By Shirley Fondiller & Barbara Nerone*	14-2551	$25.95	$22.95
☐ **The Writer's Workbook** *By Shirley Fondiller*	14-2470	23.95	20.95
☐ **Applying the Art and Science of Human Caring** *Edited by Jean Watson*	42-2647	14.95	12.50
☐ **Annual Review of Women's Health, Volume II** *Edited by Beverly McElmurry & Randy Spreen Parker*	19-2669	37.95	34.35
☐ **In Women's Experience** *Edited by Patricia Munhall*	14-2612	37.95	34.35
☐ **Health as Expanding Consciousness (2nd ed.)** *By Margaret A. Newman*	14-2626	35.95	32.35
☐ **Managing Your Career in Nursing (2nd ed.)** *By Frances Henderson & Barbara McGettigan*	14-2640	28.95	26.55
☐ **Nursing Centers: The Time Is Now** *Edited by Barbara Murphy*	41-2629	25.95	22.95

PHOTOCOPY THIS FORM TO ORDER BY MAIL OR FAX

Photocopy this coupon and send with 1) a check payable to NLN, 2) credit card information, or 3) a purchase order number to: **NLN Publications Order Unit, 350 Hudson Street, New York, NY 10014 (FAX: 212-989-3710).**

Shipping & Handling Schedule	
Order Amount	Charges
Up to $24.99	$ 3.75
25.00-49.99	5.25
50.00-74.99	6.50
75.00-99.99	7.75
100.00 and up	10.00

Subtotal: $ _____

Shipping & Handling (see chart): _____

Total: $ _____

☐ Check enclosed ☐ P.O. # _____ NLN Member # (if appl.): _____

Charge the above total to ☐ Visa ☐ MasterCard ☐ American Express

Acct. #: _____ Exp. Date: _____

Authorized Signature: _____

Name _____ Title _____

Institution _____

Address _____

City, State, Zip _____

Daytime Telephone ( ) _____ Ext. _____

The Web of Inclusion